Phonetic Approaches to Speech Production in Aphasia and Related Disorders

Phonetic Approaches to Speech Production in Aphasia and Related Disorders

Edited by John H. Ryalls, Ph.D.

Centre de Recherche du
Centre Hospitalier Côte-des-Neiges
Montreal, Quebec, Canada

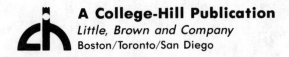

A College-Hill Publication
Little, Brown and Company
Boston/Toronto/San Diego

College-Hill Press
A Division of Little, Brown and Company (Inc.)
34 Beacon Street
Boston, Massachusetts 02108

Library of Congress Cataloging in Publication Data
Main entry under title:

Phonetic approaches to speech production in aphasia and related disorders.

"A College-Hill publication."
1. Aphasia. 2. Phonetics. I. Ryalls, John H., 1954-
[DNLM: 1. Aphasia. 2. Phonetics. 3. Speech Production Measurement.
WL 340.5 P574]
RC425.P52   1987   616.85'52   87-17051

ISBN 0-316-76371-3

C O N T E N T S

ACKNOWLEDGMENTS

I would like to thank the Max-Planck-Institute for Psycholinguistics in Nijmegen, The Netherlands, for their support in the form of a visiting fellowship in the early stages of editing this volume, as well as the Medical Research Council of Canada for a post-doctoral fellowship for the past two years. Special thanks are also in order to the members of the Laboratoire Théophile-Alajouanine for their support throughout the editing process.

P R E F A C E

It is nearly a half a century since neurologist Théophile Alajouanine published the monograph *Le syndrome de désintegration phonétique dans l'aphasie* in collaboration with psychologist André Ombredane and linguist Marguerite Durand. Many credit this collaboration with the birth of neurolinguistics in general, and it is certainly precursor to the work represented in this volume. Their formula of collaboration between neurology, psychology, and linguistics remains a model for work in this highly interdisciplinary field, and their work using Rousselot cylinders to measure acoustic characteristics of disordered speech in 1939 remains relevant today.

The advent of the digital computer for speech signal analysis has contributed to a great increase in phonetic studies of aphasia (and related disorders such as apraxia of speech and patients with right-hemisphere damage). This book assesses our present state of knowledge and provides a forum for new work in this area from different laboratories in several countries. In many ways, this volume represents the "state of the art"; however, even at the time of going to press, there are new works already in progress. Such is the on-going nature of scientific investigation. Hopefully, however, this book will serve to effectively review what phonetic approaches have taught us about speech in aphasia and related disorders, and point out the issues that future studies should address. It is directed to linguists, neuropsychologists, speech-language pathologists, and speech scientists, as well as to all students of disordered speech production.

I am especially pleased to have had the opportunity to be the catalyst for this volume, and to have been able to bring together work from various laboratories on three different continents. I would like to thank the contributors for their enthusiasm, encouragement, and willing contributions. Bill Cooper was especially helpful from the earliest stages, as was Sheila Blumstein. While it may not be appropriate to dedicate an edited volume to one person when the contributors were not specifically informed of such a dedication from the beginning, I am sure that everyone here will be happy to let me dedicate at least my editing efforts to Sheila Blumstein. This fine scholar has been a pioneer in the area of phonetic approaches to aphasia and has been a teacher of many of the contributors to this volume.

I can state without hesitation that her work and personal example have been extremely important to all in this volume. I'd like to close with these words of dedication to her:

You can date the evolving life of a mind, like the age of a tree, by the rings of friendship formed by the expanding central trunk. In the course of my life, not love or marriage so much as friendship has promoted growth.

How I Grew—Mary McCarthy
(*Vanity Fair*, March 1986, p. 134)

C O N T R I B U T O R S

Shari Baum, PhD
Department of Cognitive and Linguistic Sciences
Brown University
Providence, Rhode Island

Susan J. Behrens, PhD
Neuropsychology Program
Memorial Sloan-Kettering
1275 York Avenue
New York, New York

Sheila E. Blumstein, PhD
Department of Cognitive and Linguistic Sciences
Brown University
Providence, Rhode Island

William E. Cooper, PhD
Department of Psychology
Spense Laboratories of Psychology
University of Iowa
Iowa City, Iowa

Jack Gandour, PhD
Department of Audiology and Speech Sciences
Heavilon Hall
Purdue University
West Lafayette, Indiana

W. J. Hardcastle, PhD
Department of Linguistic Science
Faculty of Letters and Social Sciences
University of Reading
Whiteknights
Reading, Great Britain

Motonobu Itoh, PhD
Tokyo Metropolitan Institute of Gerontology
Tokyo, Japan

William Katz, PhD
Department of Psychiatry
University of California San Diego
La Jolla, California

Eric Keller, PhD
Laboratoire Théophile-Alajouanine
Centre de Recherche du C.H.C.N.
Montréal, Canada

Raymond D. Kent, PhD
Department of Communicative Disorders
University of Wisconsin-Madison
Madison, Wisconsin

Gayle V. Klouda, PhD
Department of Psychology
Spense Laboratories of Psychology
University of Iowa
Iowa City, Iowa

Malcolm R. McNeil, PhD
Department of Communicative Disorders
University of Wisconsin-Madison
Madison, Wisconsin

John H. Ryalls, PhD
Laboratoire Théophile-Alajouanine
Centre de Recherche du C.H.C.N.
Montréal, Canada

Sumiko Sasanuma, PhD
Tokyo Metropolitan Institute of Gerontology
Tokyo, Japan

Robin Seider Story
Haskins Laboratories
New Haven, Connecticut

Betty Tuller, PhD
Department of Psychology
Florida Atlantic University
Boca Raton, Florida

Wolfram Ziegler, PhD
Neuropsychological Department
Max-Planck-Institute for Psychiatry
Munich, Federal German Republic

P A R T I

Overview

C H A P T E R 1

Consonant Production Deficits in Aphasia

Sheila E. Blumstein
Shari Baum

I t is clear from both formal and informal analysis of aphasic speech that most aphasic patients exhibit deficits in the production of the sound segments of language, and in particular, the production of consonants. Interestingly, such deficits often emerge in patients with very different clinical symptomatologies and lesion sites. In-depth study of these speech production deficits has been strongly influenced and guided by the constructs of linguistic theory. For example, researchers have investigated the patterns of performance in the production of consonant *segments* and in the properties or *features* comprising these sound segments in order to explore the nature of the underlying impairments contributing to deficits in consonant production. Studies have explored the production of such attributes or features such as voicing in stop consonants, place of articulation in stop consonants, and the production of nasal and stop manner of articulation. It is worth noting that *segment* and *feature* are theoretical constructs hypothesized by linguists to be basic primitives in the sound structure of natural language.

Analyses in terms of segments and features have provided a useful heuristic in the study of speech production deficits in aphasia. In particular, early studies have shown that the phonological errors produced by aphasic patients involve very particular types of modifications to sound segments (Blumstein, 1973). These include the substitution of one sound segment for another, the loss or addition of a sound segment in an utterance, and the transposition or assimilation of sound segments that occur in neighboring environments. With respect to substitution errors, such errors are more likely to occur between sounds that share most phonetic features.

3

In the review that follows, we will consider the nature of the deficits in consonant production in aphasic patients. To this end, we will focus on studies investigating the production of consonant segments and the properties of the features comprising them. We will discuss results from studies investigating voicing in stop consonants and fricatives, contrasts of manner of articulation for nasal and stop consonants, and distinctions of place of articulation in stop consonants and fricatives. In this discussion, we will focus our attention on studies which have conducted phonetic analyses of aphasic speech. Two approaches have been taken in this vein. By far the more common approach has involved acoustic analyses of speech production. On the basis of such analyses, inferences can be made about the articulatory states that give rise to the particular acoustic patterns that emerge. An alternative approach is to conduct physiological investigations, analyzing the patterns of movement of particular parts of the articulatory system. Although it provides a direct measure of the articulatory apparatus, such research is very difficult to instrument and analyze, and, as a consequence, only a limited number of studies has been conducted. The major focus of this review will therefore be on acoustic analyses, although several physiological studies will be considered as well.

The focus on segments and features not only provides a framework for discussion of the nature of speech production deficits in aphasia, but it also allows us to consider a number of important theoretical issues. The first issue is whether all consonant segments and their associated properties are affected with speech production deficits in aphasia. In other words, is the speech output disorder a pervasive one or it selective with respect to particular aspects of speech? If it is selective, in what ways is it selective? The vulnerability of certain phonetic dimensions over others may provide important clues as to the nature of the phonetic impairments in aphasia. For example, if the phonetic disorder is primarily a temporal one, then phonetic dimensions that are primarily temporal in nature will show selective impairments. Particularly vulnerable would be voicing in initial stops and fricatives, duration of vowels as cues to postvocalic voiced and voiceless stops, as well as the intrinsic duration of fricatives, which varies as a function of place of articulation. In contrast, if the disorder is one of timing, but related to the integration or timing of independent articulators, then voicing in initial stops and fricatives as well as the production of nasal consonants would be impaired, while the production of the other parameters listed earlier should be relatively spared. And if the timing disorder is specifically limited to the relation between the supralaryngeal system and the laryngeal mechanism, then *only* the voicing of consonants will be impaired.

Similarly, the patterns of impairment should help determine whether they are primarily phonetic or phonological in nature. Linguistic theory makes a clear-cut distinction between these two levels of analysis. The phonological level is an abstract level corresponding to the selection of the phonological representation (theoretically specified in terms of features) of a lexical item. The phonetic level reflects the implementation of this abstract phonological representation, and its ultimate realization by the articulatory system. Thus, rules of the grammar specifying the full phonetic detail of the phonological representation as well as the rules of articulatory implementation and coding are represented at this level.

Turning to the potential dichotomy between phonological and phonetic disorders in aphasia, a phonological impairment would reflect an inability to appropriately access and/or select a phonological representation of a particular lexical item or utterance. Such a deficit would result in a correctly articulated but incorrectly planned sound structure, e.g., pot → [bat]. In contrast, a phonetic disorder would reflect an inability to appropriately translate the phonological representation into its correct articulatory realization. Such a deficit could result in a correctly planned utterance which is articulated incorrectly, e.g., pot → [p^{hh}at].

There are a number of ways to explore whether the basis of production deficits in aphasia is primarily phonetic or phonological. Perhaps the most obvious is to explore the acoustic patterns corresponding to the production of particular phonetic attributes to determine whether the patterns of the patients deviate in any way from the acoustic patterns of normal subjects. If they do, the issue is to specify and quantify the nature of the deviations in order to determine what articulatory configurations could produce such acoustic patterns. Systematic deviations suggest an impairment in the instantiation or realization of a phonetic feature. Even productions that sound perceptually as though they are sound substitutions, e.g., [p] → [b], could be analyzed in this way to determine whether a subset of substitution errors or even most substitution errors are in fact extreme phonetic distortions rather than true phonological errors.

Another way of exploring whether the basis of speech production deficits is phonetic or phonological in nature is to focus on particular acoustic attributes corresponding to phonetic features or dimensions. There are a number of acoustic parameters that may serve either a phonological or phonetic function. For example, duration of the frication noise is a critical attribute distinguishing voiced from voiceless fricatives. In this case, duration has a constrastive function, distinguishing one sound segment from another, and it thus serves as a phonological feature. Duration also serves a phonetic role in fricative consonants—each fricative has its own characteristic or intrinsic duration with [f θ] in English being shorter in duration than [s š]. Because this duration parameter characterizes a property of these fricatives, yet is not used in the language system phonemically to distinguish among the class of fricatives, duration in this case is properly a phonetic feature. It is possible to explore whether aphasic patients show contrasts between the use of duration as a contrastive versus an intrinsic property of consonant production. Such results should help determine whether the patient's deficit is primarily phonological or phonetic in nature.

While it may be a useful heuristic to study consonant production in terms of sound segments and the features that comprise them, segments are not produced in the stream of speech as "beads on a string," i.e., as individual, independent units, isolated from the sounds around them. Rather, the sounds of speech exert considerable influence on each other. For example, the production of [s] in the syllables [si] and [su] is affected by the neighboring vowel sounds. The speaker will round his or her lips while producing [s] in anticipation of the following rounded vowel [u], while such rounding does not occur in the production of [s] in the environment of [i]. Such *coarticulatory* influences affect the resultant acoustic patterns of the production of [s]. Ultimately, the sound stream of speech is produced by timing relations and the integration of motor movements that go well beyond the production of individual consonant segments and the features comprising them. Consequently, another aspect of studying deficits in consonant production in aphasia is to investigate the nature of coarticulation. Such study will provide further critical information on the basis of the speech production deficits in aphasia. At issue is whether patients show the same type of coarticulatory effects as do normals, and whether any obtained impairments reflect a limitation on the number of planning units that can be programmed (hence a phonological disorder), or the implementation of such units in the production of syllables or words (hence a phonetic disorder). Several chapters of this volume are dedicated to this very important issue, and hence, we will not further consider coarticulation in aphasia.

In our review, we will consider the nature of consonant production in different types of aphasic patients. Although most studies have focussed on the speech production impairments of Broca's aphasics and patients with apraxia of speech, it is essential to understand which patterns of impairment are selective with respect to these types of patients and which patterns of impairment are not. Only in this way, will we ultimately be able to determine the neurological mechanisms that contribute to speech-production deficits in aphasia. Consequently, we will also examine speech production in other types of aphasic patients including Wernicke's aphasics.

One further point regarding subject selection deserves mention. The speech of patients diagnosed as having Broca's aphasia, apraxia of speech, and dysarthria have all been studied with respect to the production of consonants (cf. Buckingham, 1981). In the present review, we will not discuss dysarthric speech, as it is a deficit characterized by muscular weakness or incoordination, rather than a higher-order or more abstract articulatory implementation deficit. The results of studies investigating the speech of patients diagnosed as Broca's aphasics and those with apraxia of speech have been, for the most part, indistinguishable, and, in fact, there is some debate in the literature whether these two syndromes are in fact distinct (Lesser, 1978; Buckingham, 1981). Consequently, for the purposes of this review, it is assumed that the articulatory disorder of Broca's aphasia corresponds roughly to the impairment known as apraxia of speech, and will be treated as comparable disorders. However, the patients will be referred to in terms of the diagnoses made by authors of the individual studies discussed, and we will note any results that hinge on potential differences in classification.

Throughout the following discussion, an attempt will be made to synthesize the data presented into a coherent description of the various speech production impairments of aphasic patients and their underlying deficits. At the outset of each section, the articulatory and/or acoustic parameters characterizing normal production of the given phonetic attribute will be briefly reviewed. The phonetic parameter or feature that has received the most attention in the literature is voicing, and it is with this feature that this review will begin.

VOICING

There are a number of parameters that contribute to voicing contrasts in consonants. For stops consonants, the parameter that has received the most attention is voice-onset time. Voice-onset time (VOT) reflects the timing relation between the release of a stop consonant and the onset of voicing (i.e., vocal fold vibration). Voiceless consonants have longer VOTs than voiced consonants. In English, voiceless consonants such as [p t k] have VOT values that range from 40 ms to 100 ms or more. In contrast, voiced consonants such as [b d g] are produced with VOT values with no voicing lag or short-lag VOTs, thus ranging between 0 and approximately 20 ms, or they are produced with prevoicing. In the case of prevoicing, voicing begins prior to the release of the stop closure. Typically, when voiced and voiceless stop consonants are produced by normal subjects in initial position in citation form (i.e. as words or syllables spoken in isolation), two non-overlapping distributions of VOT occur (Lisker & Abramson, 1964). While there are some changes in these distributions with age, the distinction between the voiced and voiceless categories is still maintained, and for the most part, there is not overlap between voiced and voiceless categories (Itoh et al., 1982; Shewan, Leeper, & Booth, 1982; Sweeting & Baken, 1982).

It is worth emphasizing that voice-onset time is only one of several parameters distinguishing voiced and voiceless stops in initial position. Voiced stop consonants not only have shorter VOTs than do voiceless consonants, but they also have shorter and weaker bursts (Lisker & Abramson, 1964; Pickett, 1980).

In final position, stop consonants in English are distinguished by a number of parameters. These include the duration of the stop closure, the presence or absence of voicing during the closure interval, and the duration of the preceding vowel (Raphael, 1972; Port, 1976). For final voiced stops, the closure interval is shorter than that for voiceless stops, voicing is present during the closure interval, and the duration of the preceding vowel is longer, e.g., *bead* [bi:d] vs. *beat* [bit]. Normal subjects appear to produce two nonoverlapping distributions of vowel durations with the duration of the vowels preceding voiced stops ranging from approximately 200–400 ms, and voiceless stops ranging from approximately 100–225 ms (cf., Duffy & Gawle, 1984; Tuller, 1984).

Similar to stop consonants, a parameter of duration distinguishes initial voiced and voiceless fricative consonants. The duration of the frication noise for voiceless fricatives is longer than that for voiced fricatives. Although the overall mean of the frication noise may be shorter for voiced compared to voiceless fricatives, preliminary data suggest that there is considerable overlap in the duration of voiced and voiceless fricative consonants in normals (Baum & Blumstein, 1987b).

What is of particular interest for our consideration of consonant production in aphasic patients is that there are a number of different duration parameters that contribute to voicing contrasts in consonants: VOT distinguishes initial voiced and voiceless stops, vowel duration distinguishes final voiced and voiceless stops, and the duration of the fricative noise distinguishes voiced and voiceless fricatives. The patterns of impairment in aphasia may help determine whether the voicing feature, in particular, is compromised. If this were the case, impairments should emerge for the three different measures of voicing. Alternatively, only particular parameters of voicing may be impaired. Let us review the evidence.

A fairly large number of studies have been conducted to determine whether aphasic patients demonstrate the VOT patterns exhibited by normals. The first studies to explore this question were conducted by Blumstein and her colleagues (Blumstein et al., 1977; 1980). Results of these studies showed differential patterns of performance in the production of VOT as a function of type of aphasia. In particular, Wernicke's aphasics showed a VOT distribution similar to normals in that they maintained the category distinction between voiced and voiceless stops, and there was minimal, if any, overlap between the VOT boundaries between the voiced and voiceless stops. Nevertheless, not all of the productions of the Wernicke's aphasics were normal. They did produce target voiced and voiceless stops whose VOT values fell within the range of the alternate phonetic category, e.g., a target [d] having a VOT of 100 ms or a target [t] having a VOT of 10 ms.

The distribution of VOTs of the anterior and Broca's aphasics were in sharp contrast to those of Wernicke's aphasics. These patients were unable to maintain the category distinction between voiced and voiceless stops. That is, there was overlap in the VOT distribution for the production of voiced and voiceless stops. In addition, similar to the Wernicke's aphasics, these patients also produced utterances that fell within the range of the alternate phonetic category.

The results have been replicated in a number of studies using other aphasic patients (Hoit-Dalgaard, Murry, & Kopp, 1983; Shewan, Leeper, & Booth, 1984; Tuller, 1984) and in languages other than English, including Japanese and Thai (Itoh, et al., 1982; Gandour & Dardarananda, 1984). Broca's aphasics (Shewan et al., 1984; Tuller, 1984) and patients with apraxia of speech (Hoit-Dalgaard et al., 1983; Itoh et al., 1982) have shown overlap of VOT for voiced and voiceless tokens, and Wernicke's aphasics (Tuller, 1984) have generally maintained the distinction between these two categories.

Nevertheless, conflicting findings have been reported for conduction aphasics. Consistent with claims that there are two distinct anatomical patterns underlying conduction aphasia (Benson et al., 1973; Damasio & Damasio, 1983), Blumstein and colleagues (1980) found two different patterns of VOT among the conduction aphasics tested—one pattern was similar to that obtained for Broca's aphasics, and the other was similar to that obtained for Wernicke's aphasics. Itoh and colleagues (1982) challenged these findings reporting that the 2 conduction aphasics that they tested had VOT distributions similar to those of Wernicke's aphasics. In contrast, Shewan and colleagues (1984) found no difference in VOT patterns between the Broca's and conduction aphasics that they tested. Clearly more research is needed to determine why these particular disparities emerged. A likely explanation is that the different lesion sites contributing to the conduction aphasia symptomatology produce potential differences in patterns of consonant production (cf. Blumstein et al., 1980; Damasio & Damasio, 1983).

Of particular interest is a study by Gandour and Dardarananda (1984) who explored VOT production in a group of Thai aphasic subjects. In Thai, there is a three-way VOT distinction amoung voiced unaspirated, voiceless unaspirated, and voiceless aspirated stop consonants. Voiced stops are prevoiced, voiceless unaspirated stops have a short-lag VOT, and voiceless aspirated stops have a long-lag VOT. Broca's aphasics and global aphasics showed overlap between prevoiced and voiceless unaspirated stops, as well as overlap between voiceless unaspirated and voiceless aspirated stops. That is, they were unable to maintain the category distinction in this three-valued system. In contrast, Wernicke's, transcortical motor, and conduction aphasics showed minimal impairments.

The basic conclusions concerning VOT production in aphasia have been the same in all of these studies. It has been suggested that Wernicke's aphasics have primarily a phonological impairment in that they produce a voiced or voiceless stop consonant that is phonetically correct but which may be phonologically incorrect. In contrast, Broca's aphasics and patients with apraxia of speech seem to have primarily a phonetic disorder affecting the articulatory implementation of voiced and voiceless stops. It is less clear from these results whether Broca's have a phonological impairment as well. It is impossible to determine whether those VOT productions that fall in the range of the alternate phonetic category reflect gross phonetic distortions or phonological substitutions. Researchers in the field are divided on this issue, and alternative procedures will be necessary to determine which is the correct interpretation.

Even though Broca's aphasics clearly have an impairment in the temporal coordination of the release of the stop closure and the onset of vocal fold vibration, it is not possible to determine on the basis of the VOT studies alone whether the deficit displayed by Broca's aphasics reflects a pervasive phonetic disorder affecting, e.g., all phonetic parameters of voicing or whether it reflects a more selective timing impairment. To explore this issue, it is necessary to explore the other duration parameters contributing to voicing in final voiced and voiceless stop consonants and initial fricative consonants. Let us turn to the results of these studies.

Results of investigations of vowel duration preceding voiced and voiceless stop consonants in CVC words, e.g., *beat* versus *bead*, provide some interesting new insights into production deficits in aphasia. Duffy and Gawle (1984) measured vowel duration in CVC utterances produced by aphasics with and without apraxia of speech. Results of their analyses indicated that although the absolute duration of the vowels was shorter in these patients, and the vowel durations were produced with greater variability than found with normals, they nonetheless maintained the vowel duration distinction as a cue to stop consonant voicing. Importantly, they not only varied vowel duration as a function of postvocalic voicing of the stop consonants, but they did so to a degree comparable to that of normals. Similar findings were obtained by Baum and Blumstein (1987a) for a group of Broca's aphasics. These results suggest that the impairment of patients with apraxia of speech and Broca's aphasia is not selective with respect to the feature of voicing, as one phonetic parameter of this feature, VOT, is relatively impaired, whereas another phonetic parameter, vowel duration, is relatively spared.

Tuller (1984) explored this question more directly by comparing the production of VOT and vowel duration in the same patients. Her analysis procedures were based on the degree to which the patients maintained a bimodal distribution in their productions of VOT and vowel duration. Her results showed that there was no necessary relation between the nature or type of distribution in any one subject for these two parameters. Thus, the basis of the disorder for these patients seems to be more properly characterized as a phonetic one, affecting durational patterns of speech, and particularly the timing relation between two independent articulators (e.g., the tongue or lips and the larynx).

All of these studies compared the performance of apraxic or Broca's patients with other aphasic patients. The other patients were clinically diverse, consisting of Wernicke's aphasics (Tuller, 1984; Baum & Blumstein, 1987a) and a hetergeneous group of patients who were nonapraxic (Duffy & Gawle, 1984). Interestingly, the performance of these patients was not normal. They also showed overall shorter mean vowel durations and greater variability (Duffy & Gawle, 1984). And although the Wernicke's aphasics tested by Tuller (1984) tended to have more bimodal distributions than the Broca's aphasics she tested, this was not the case for all of the Wernicke's aphasics tested. Finally, Baum & Blumstein (1987a) found that although both Broca's and Wernicke's aphasics maintained the distinction between final voiced and voiceless stops as a function of vowel duration, the performance of the two groups did not differ from each other. These results suggest that other aphasic types, and in particular Wernicke's aphasics, may also have subtle phonetic impairments. This suggestion was first made by Blumstein et al. (1980) who had noted in their analyses that some Wernicke's aphasics showed evidence for phonetic impairments in the production of initial voiced and voiceless stops. The implications of these findings will be discussed as other phonetic parameters are considered.

The final phonetic parameter for voicing that will be reviewed is the duration of the frication noise as a cue to voiced and voiceless fricative consonants. Results have shown that the duration measures for Broca's aphasics, patients with apraxia of speech, and Wernicke's aphasics are similar to those found for normals (Code & Ball, 1982; Kent & Rosenbek, 1983; Harmes et al., 1984; Baum & Blumstein, 1987a). In particular, voiceless fricatives tend to have longer durations than do voiced fricatives. Nevertheless, all of these studies have noted that both Broca's aphasics and patients with apraxia of speech have difficulty in producing voiced fricatives. These consonants are produced with inconsistent voicing throughout the duration of the frication noise. In fact, the Broca's aphasics studied by Code and Ball (1982) showed virtually no evidence of voicing during this interval. Kent and Rosenbek (1983) noted in their study of 7 patients with apraxia of speech that the onset of frication did not consistently coincide with the onset of voicing in initial voiceless fricatives.

All of the data gathered in the analyses of the duration parameters contributing to voicing in consonant production suggest that Broca's aphasics and patients with apraxia of speech have a deficit in temporal control and coordination. Nevertheless, their impairment does not simply reflect an inability to appropriately control duration since vowel duration as a phonetic parameter distinguishing final voiced and voiceless stops is relatively spared as is frication noise duration distinguishing initial voiced and voiceless fricatives. Instead, the patients seem to have particular difficulty in the timing relation between two independent articulators and, in the case of both initial stops and fricatives, in the timing relation between gestures of the supralaryngeal vocal tract and gestures of the larynx.

Potential phonetic impairments attributed to Wernicke's aphasics are less clear-cut. The fact that they show some subtle impairments in the production of VOT and vowel duration suggests that they, too, have a speech production disorder that may affect articulatory implementation. Nevertheless, the nature of the speech output of these patients, as well as the patterns of impairments, reviewed thus far suggest that their difficulties are qualitatively different from those found for Broca's aphasics and patients with apraxia of speech.

Studies of manner of articulation in aphasia will be discussed next in an attempt to further refine our characterization of the consonant production deficits of aphasic patients.

MANNER OF ARTICULATION

Very few studies have actually focussed on the phonetic analysis of contrasts of manner of articulation. A hierarchy of difficulty in the production of various consonant types has been established based on the patterns of errors produced by aphasic patients. Specifically, it has been shown that stops and nasals are easier to produce than both fricatives and affricates, and that singleton consonants are easier to produce than clusters (Shankweiler & Harris, 1966; Blumstein, 1973; Trost & Canter, 1974).

The one study that has contrasted the production of manner of articulation distinctions experimentally focussed on the nasal-stop distinction. The timing of velar movements is critical to the production of nasal consonants. In particular, for nasal consonants, the velar opening is coincident with the closure in the oral cavity corresponding to a particular place of articulation, e.g., [m] or [n], and it closes rapidly in some 20-odd ms after the release of the closure in the oral cavity. In contrast, in the production of stop consonants, the velum is closed throughout the stop closure and release into the following vowel. Anticipatory and carryover coarticulation effects of the velar opening may be present, but apparently do not extend over a very long period of time (Itoh et al., 1979; 1980).

Using fiberscopic and x-ray microbeam examination, Itoh and colleagues (1979; 1980) explored the timing of the velar opening prior to the production of a nasal consonant embedded in a carrier phrase, e.g., [denee], in the speech of a single apraxic patient. Although the general successional patterns of velar gestures approximated those for normals, they found variability in the patterns of velar movements. Their patient tended to lower his velum earlier than normal, often at the beginning of the first vowel. Moreover, the patterns of velar closing were less consistent. Further, they found deficits in the timing relations between velar lowering and the lip and tongue movements for the production of [n]. Although they did not measure directly the timing relation of the tongue tip at the release of the closure at the alveolar ridge with velar lowering in the production of [n], Itoh and colleagues (1979; 1980) suggest that their apraxic patient had difficulty in the timing and coordination of velar maneuvers simultaneous to the production of a consonantal constriction.

In contrast, the two Wernicke's aphasics tested (Itoh et al., 1983) displayed patterns of velar movements more in accord with normal subjects. The Wernicke's patients nevertheless, did produce errors in the production of nasals, sometimes substituting nasals and stops for each other. Itoh and colleagues (1983) analyzed these productions and found that the patterns of velar movement corresponded to those expected for the alternate category. That is, errors were not due to inexact velar movements, but rather to movements appropriate to another phoneme. Consequently, they concluded that while apraxic patients have an articulatory timing impairment, Wernicke's aphasics have a phonological or selection impairment.

It is of interest to explore the production of other manners of articulation to determine whether they too are impaired in the speech production of aphasic patients. Unlike nasal and stop consonants, fricatives are produced with a constriction rather than a closure in the oral cavity, and this constriction must be maintained over some 100 ms or more. Moreover, fricatives with different places of articulation have different intrinsic durations. [s] and [š] are consistently longer than are [f] and [θ] in initial position in the speech production of normal subjects. Acoustic analyses of Broca's aphasics' ability to produce fricative consonants have shown that surprisingly the patterns of production of Broca's aphasics do not differ from normals. In particular, Harmes and colleagues (1984) showed in their analysis of the production of [s] and [z] by four Broca's aphasics that they maintained normal control of duration of [s] and [z] across a number of phonetic contexts. And Baum and Blumstein (1987a) showed that Broca's aphasics maintained the intrinsic durations inherent to the different places of articulation of the voiceless fricatives [f θ s š].

Thus, the parameters explored to date for the production of fricative manner of articulation suggest that Broca's aphasics are similar to normals. Clearly, a great deal more research is needed exploring in-depth the acoustic parameters associated with the production of manner of articulation in consonants. However, within the limited set of data available, the results suggest that not all properties associated with the production of manner of articulation are impaired. Thus, the articulatory impairment of Broca's or apraxic patients does not seem to be pervasive with respect to manner of articulation categories, but rather seems to be relatively selective with respect to the articulatory dimensions associated with particular manners of articulation.

PLACE OF ARTICULATION

Production of place of articulation is a critical parameter to consider in the investigation of speech production deficits in aphasia. First, place of articulation errors are among the most common types of errors produced by aphasic patients (Blumstein, 1973). Moreover, unlike the acoustic parameters discussed for voicing and manner of articulation that are primarily temporal or durational in nature, the acoustic parameters corresponding to place of articulation are primarily spectral in nature. That is, the primary attributes distinguishing different places of articulation turn on the relative distribution of energy in the spectrum.

A number of measurement procedures have been developed in the normal literature for the acoustic analysis of place of articulation in stop consonants. One measure developed by Stevens and Blumstein (Stevens & Blumstein, 1978; Blumstein & Stevens, 1979) explored the gross shape of the onset spectrum. They found that the spectral properties measured in the first 20-odd ms at consonantal release uniquely distinguished labial, alveolar, and velar places of articulation in English stop consonants. These properties emerged independent of the vowel context and speaker. Labial consonants had a diffuse-falling or diffuse-flat spectral shape. Alveolar consonants had a diffuse-rising shape. And velar consonants had a compact spectrum shape.

In order to quantify these observations, Blumstein and Stevens (1979) developed a set of three templates, one for each of the labial, alveolar, and velar places of articulation. Using the same template-matching procedures, Shinn and Blumstein (1983) investigated the spectral characteristics of place of articulation in five aphasic patients—four Broca's and one Wernicke's— and compared them to the results obtained by Blumstein and Stevens (1979) for their six normal subjects.

Results can be summarized as follows. In general, the spectral properties of the stop consonants produced by the aphasic patients were similar to normals. These results were particularly striking for stimuli that were consistently perceived correctly for place of articulation by normal listeners. For stimuli that were not perceived consistently by listeners, the spectral properties fit the templates less well. Nevertheless, on balance, the results suggested that the Broca's aphasics were able to reach the correct articulatory configuration for place of articulation.

Of particular interest is that the data used in this study were a subset of those used in the Blumstein and colleagues (1980) study of VOT. The results of the VOT study showed that the Broca's aphasics were not able to maintain the distinction between the voiced and voiceless phonetic categories. These same utterances, analyzed acoustically in terms of their spectral properties for place of articulation, did not show the striking impairments for Broca's aphasics that the VOT analysis revealed.

Nevertheless, Broca's aphasics were not entirely normal in their productions, and they tended to have the greatest difficulty in producing alveolar consonants. In particular, the spectral properties of the alveolar stop consonants produced by Broca's aphasics had much less high frequency energy than normally found. Two potential problems were suggested to account for this pattern of productions. Both concern the nature of the source characteristics of the articulatory mechanism.

According to the source-filter theory of speech production (Fant, 1960), the acoustic characteristics of speech sounds involve the complex interaction of the source of energy and the filter function. For human speech sounds, the source of energy is provided at the larynx and/or at the source of constriction in the vocal tract. The supralaryngeal vocal tract acts as an acoustic filter, suppressing the transfer of energy at certain frequencies and letting more energy through at other frequencies. Changes in the shape of the supralaryngeal vocal tract can alter the filter function. If there is a change in the nature of the source characteristics, there may be a modification of the obtained spectral characteristics of the sounds.

The spectral patterns of alveolar consonants produced by Broca's aphasics suggest a change in the laryngeal source, and as we have noted in the analysis of voicing, these patients have particular difficulties in laryngeal control. A second problem may be in the nature of the source at the constriction in the vocal tract. In particular, a failure to produce a complete closure in the production of stop consonants could result in the coupling of the front and back cavity resonances producing the types of spectral patterns that were observed.

Taken together, these results suggest that the patient knows the target place of articulation, in that he can get his articulators into the correct configuration for place of articulation. Nevertheless, the dynamic aspects of articulatory control seem to be impaired. That is, the Broca's aphasics' difficulties with the source characteristics of speech sounds implicate impairments in the integration of motor movements over time, as exemplified by the nature of the release characteristics of the sound, and impairments in the integration of articulatory movements in the vocal tract, as exemplified by laryngeal control. Since these deviations reflect modifications of the vocal tract configuration, problems with place of articulation seem to reflect phonetic, i.e., articulatory implementation, impairments, rather than phonological planning errors.

Similar conclusions were made by Harmes and colleagues (1984) in their study of fricative production in Broca's aphasics. They conducted spectral analyses of the production of [s] and [z] spoken in different environments by four Broca's aphasics. Similar to the findings for the production of alveolar stop consonants, they found spectral differences between the utterances of their aphasics and normal controls. The Broca's aphasics produced lower spectral cut-off frequencies than normals; a downward shift of the two largest spectral peaks; a reduction in the peakiness of the spectrum; and a downward shifting of the power band-width of the center frequencies and upper cut-off frequencies. Harmes and colleagues (1984) suggest that this pattern of results indicates that Broca's patients generally can produce the correct place of articulation, but have poor articulatory control, thus making many errors of *imprecision* in their attempts to produce an anterior lingual articulation. Consistent with this view are recent results of Baum and Blumstein (1987a) who showed that Broca's aphasics maintain the intrinsic durations characteristic of the different places of articulation for the voiceless fricatives [f ө s š]. Thus, Broca's aphasics generally approximate the "correct" place of articulation, despite a lack of articulatory precision.

While it seems clear that Broca's aphasics have phonetic impairments in the production of place of articulation, there is also a suggestion that they make phonological errors as well. Shinn and Blumstein (1983) noted that in addition to the phonetic impairments that emerged in their Broca's aphasics, there was a subset of errors produced by both the Broca's aphasics and the Wernicke's patient that seemed to reflect phonological errors rather than phonetic errors. In particular, the phonemic paraphasias that involved place of articulation (e.g., [d] → [b]) were acoustically analyzed to determine if the acoustic properties reflected the spectral characteristics of the substituted sound or alternatively distorted characteristics of either the target sound or the substituted sound. Results indicated that these paraphasias consistently maintained the spectral characteristics of the substituted sound. That is, they were good *phonetic* exemplars of the substituted category. Unlike voicing errors (as measured by VOT) in which it is unclear whether a voicing substitution reflects a true substitution or a distortion along the voicing continuum, a place of articulation error cannot reflect the same type of "distortion" along a continuum. The spectral properties that coincide with different places of articulation reflect completely different articulatory gestures, not continuous variations along a single articulatory parameter. Thus, Broca's aphasics seem to produce both phonological and phonetic errors in the production of place of articulation in stop consonants.

CONCLUSION

In this chapter, the authors have considered patterns of consonant production as a means of assessing the nature of speech production deficits in aphasia. The constellation of impairments shown by Broca's aphasics and patients with apraxia of speech clearly implicates a phonetic disorder. In particular, analysis of the acoustic patterns corresponding to the production of voicing in stop consonants and fricative consonants, and the production of nasal consonants, revealed that these patients are unable to normally articulate these speech sounds. Perhaps more importantly, these patterns suggest that the nature of the phonetic disorder is of a very particular kind. The patients' phonetic disorder does not seem to be grounded in the failure to instantiate particular phonetic features, but rather in the inability to implement particular types of articulatory gestures or articulatory parameters. If the phonetic disorder had reflected an impairment in the instantiation of a particular feature, then Broca's aphasics should have shown deficits in the production of the various acoustic parameters contributing to voicing. However, results indicated that voicing in initial stops and fricatives was affected, whereas the production of vowel duration as a cue to postvocalic voicing was relatively normal, as was fricative duration as a cue to initial voiced and voiceless fricatives. Thus, the articulatory implementation of the voicing feature was not compromised, but particular instantiations of that feature were compromised—namely, those that involve the temporal coordination of the release of a closure or a constriction and the onset of vocal cord vibration.

It is clear from data that the Broca's aphasics and patients with apraxia of speech have impairments with the articulatory implementation of temporal parameters. However, the data also indicate that the basis of this disorder is not simply temporal in nature, but, in effect, is more specific than that. In particular, the patients do not demonstrate impairments with all temporal or durational parameters of speech. The duration of vowels as a cue to postvocalic voicing, the duration of the fricative noise as a cue to voicing, and the intrinsic duration of the fricative noise that varies among the voiceless fricatives of English are all maintained by Broca's aphasics and patients with apraxia of speech. These patients seem to be particularly vulnerable to those phonetic parameters requiring the temporal integration of the movement of two independent articulators. Thus, not only is the voicing of stop consonants and fricative consonants impaired (reflecting the timing relation between the release of the stop closure or constriction and the onset of voicing), but also the production of nasal consonants (reflecting the timing relation between the release of the oral closure and the closing of the velum).

This timing problem may be a manifestation of a broader problem in the dynamics of speech production, i.e., the integration of articulatory movements from one phonetic segment to another as well as the integration of articulatory movements for a single phonetic segment. Thus, Kent and Rosenbek (1983) have shown extreme lengthening in the formant transitions of consonants, reflecting a difficulty in integrating articulatory movements from the articulatory gestures for a consonant into those for a vowel. Moreover, they also showed that although the patients had problems with the control of timing and coordination, the acoustic manifestations of this problem varied from individual to individual. And while patients with Broca's aphasia seem to be able to get their articulators into the correct configuration for the production of place of articulation, or at least seem to "know" where their articulators need to go, they demonstrate great imprecision in getting there. These findings were particularly evident in the production of fricative consonants.

Finally, it is also clear that the laryngeal system itself is impaired in Broca's and apraxia of speech patients. This is evident not just from the analysis of those parameters involving the production of voicing, but also from the analysis of the spectral patterns derived for the production of place of articulation in stop consonants. Thus, it seems to be the case that these patients have particular difficulty in the control and timing of laryngeal gestures. These difficulties will affect not only voicing, but also those parameters that rely on the interaction of the laryngeal system with the supralaryngeal vocal tract system.

While the nature of the speech production deficit in Broca's and apraxia of speech patients seems to be primarily phonetic in nature, these patients seem to display phonological impairments as well. Those voicing errors in stop consonant production which reflect the production of VOT values corresponding to the alternate phonetic category could either be selection or implementation errors. However, place of articulation errors produced by Broca's patients do seem to derive from errors of selection, i.e., the substitution of the wrong place of articulation rather than implementation. There are many other types of phonological errors produced by Broca's aphasics that would also seem to be difficult to characterize as primarily due to articulatory implementation errors. Such errors include metathesis errors, e.g., degrees → [gədriz], and regressive assimilation errors, e.g., roast beef → [rof bif].

As to Wernicke's aphasics, nearly all evidence points to the fact that the speech production disorder of these patients is primarily phonological in nature. The acoustic analysis of the various phonetic parameters reveals that on balance these patients maintain patterns similar to normals. Nevertheless, a number of studies have suggested a subtle phonetic impairment in the production of consonants in these patients. In particular, acoustic analyses reveal that they show an increased variability in the articulatory implementation of a number of phonetic parameters. This variability is manifested in the production of the duration of the fricative noise for fricative consonants and by greater variability in the production of vowel duration as a cue to postvocalic voicing. Moreover, even some Wernicke's display abnormal VOT and vowel duration distributions (cf. Tuller, 1984). Similar findings of greater variability have emerged for these patients in the production of vowels (Ryalls, 1986).

What is not clear is the nature of the impairment contributing to this pattern of performance. One possibility is that it reflects a general brain-damage effect either subsequent to damage to the left dominant hemisphere or perhaps even to the right hemisphere. Alternatively, it could reflect the fact that posterior areas projecting to the motor/articulatory system are damaged, or the auditory feedback system contributing to normal speech production is impaired. At this point, these suggestions are merely speculative and a great deal more research is required to determine what might contribute to this subtle phonetic impairment.

In closing, it is worth emphasizing that, in general, the results of the studies discussed in this chapter represent a conservative estimate of the speech production impairments in aphasic patients, and in particular, in Broca's and apraxia of speech patients. Most studies to date have explored the production of consonants in citation form and in relatively simple (i.e., unmarked) phonetic contexts. Presumably, further impairments would be revealed in studies exploring consonant production in continuous speech and in more complex environments, e.g., consonant clusters. Although some research has been conducted in this vein (Kent & Rosenbek, 1983; Harmes et al., 1984), more detailed studies are necessary to determine the limits of the production deficits of aphasic patients and to ascertain whether impairments in other phonetic parameters will emerge. Moreover, many more phonetic parameters need to be explored and potential disorders in implementation need to be quantified. Such parameters include the different manners of articulation such as stops, affricates, glides, and liquids, and the different places of articulation across these different manners of articulation. Finally, it would also be of great value to begin to chart speech production impairments in relation to the underlying neuroanatomy. Only then can we begin to map out the mechanisms contributing to normal speech production. This chapter thus represents only a beginning in the challenging effort to understand the nature of speech production deficits in aphasia.

ACKNOWLEDGMENT

This research was supported in part by Grants NS22282 to Brown University and NS06209 to the Boston University School of Medicine.

REFERENCES

Baum, S., & Blumstein, S. (1987a). Temporal dimensions of consonant and vowel production: An acoustic analysis of aphasic speech (in preparation).

Baum, S., & Blumstein, S. (1987b). Preliminary observations on the use of duration as a cue to syllable-initial fricative consonant voicing in English (*Journal of the Acoustical Society of America*), in press.

Benson, D.F., Sheremata, W.A., Bouchard, R., Segarra, J.M., Price, D., & Geschwind, N. (1973). Conduction aphasia: A clinicopathological study. *Archives of Neurology, 28,* 339–346.

Blumstein, S. (1973). *A phonological investigation of aphasic speech.* The Hague: Mouton.

Blumstein, S., Cooper, W., Goodglass, H., Statlender, S., & Gottlieb, J. (1980). Production deficits in aphasia: A voice-onset time analysis. *Brain and Language, 9,* 153–170.

Blumstein, S., Cooper, W., Zurif, E., & Caramazza, A. (1977). The perception and production of voice-onset time in aphasia. *Neuropsychologia, 15,* 371–383.

Blumstein, S., & Stevens, K. (1979). Acoustic invariance in speech production: Evidence for measurements of the spectral characteristics of stop consonants. *Journal of the Acoustical Society of America, 66,* 1001–1017.

Buckingham, H. (1981). Explanations for the concept of apraxia of speech. In M.T. Sarno, (Ed.), *Acquired aphasia.* New York: Academic Press.

Code, C., & Ball, M. (1982). Fricative production in Broca's aphasia: A spectrographic analysis. *Journal of Phonetics, 10,* 325–331.

Damasio, A., & Damasio, H. (1983). Localization of lesions in conduction aphasia. In A. Kertesz, (Ed.), *Localization in neuropsychology.* New York: Academic Press.

Duffy, J., & Gawle, C. (1984). Apraxic speakers' vowel duration in consonant-vowel-consonant syllables. In J. Rosenbek, M. McNeil, & A. Aronson, (Eds.), *Apraxia of speech.* San Diego: College-Hill Press.

Fant, G. (1960). *Acoustic theory of speech production.* The Hague: Mouton.

Gandour, J., & Dardarananda, R. (1984). Voice onset time in aphasia: Thai, II. Production. *Brain and Language, 23,* 177–205.

Harmes, S., Daniloff, R., Hoffman, P., Lewis, J., Kramer, M., & Absher, R. (1984). Temporal and articulatory control of fricative articulation by speakers with Broca's aphasia. *Journal of Phonetics, 12,* 367–385.

Hoit-Dalgaard, J., Murry, T., & Kopp, H. (1983). Voice onset time production and perception in apraxic subjects. *Brain and Language, 20,* 329–339.

Itoh, M., & Sasanuma, S. (1983). Velar movements during speech in two Wernicke aphasic patients. *Brain and Language, 19,* 283–292.

Itoh, M., Sasanuma, S., Hirose, H., Yoshioka, H., & Ushijima, T. (1980). Abnormal articulatory dynamics in a patient with apraxia of speech. *Brain and Language, 11,* 66–75.

Itoh, M., Sasanuma, S., Tatsumi, I., Murakami, S., Fukusako, Y., & Suzuki, T. (1982). Voice onset time characteristics in apraxia of speech. *Brain and Language, 17,* 193–210.

Itoh, M., Sasanuma, S., & Ushijima, T. (1979). Velar movements during speech in a patient with apraxia of speech. *Brain and Language, 7,* 227–239.

Kent, R., & Rosenbek, J. (1983). Acoustic patterns of apraxia of speech. *Journal of Speech and Hearing Research, 26,* 231–248.

Lesser, R. (1978). *Linguistic investigations of aphasia.* New York: Elsevier.

Lisker, L., & Abramson, A. (1964). A cross-language study of voicing in initial stops: Acoustic measurements. *Word, 20,* 384–422.

Pickett, J. (1980). *The sounds of speech communication.* Baltimore, MD: University Park Press.

Port, R. (1976). *The influence of speaking tempo on the duration of stressed vowel and medial stop in English trochee words* (Unpublished doctoral dissertation, University of Connecticut).

Raphael, L. (1972). Preceding vowel duration as a cue to the perception of the voicing characteristic of word-final consonants in American English. *Journal of the Acoustical Society of America, 51*, 1296–1303.

Ryalls, J. (1986). An acoustic study of vowel production in aphasia. *Brain and Language, 29*, 48–67.

Shankweiler, D., & Harris, K. (1966). An experimental approach to the problem of articulation in aphasia. *Cortex, 2*, 277–292.

Shewan, C., Leeper, H., & Booth, J. (1984). An analysis of voice onset time (VOT) in aphasic and normal subjects. In J. Rosenbek, M. McNeil, & A. Aronson, (Eds.), *Apraxia of speech.* San Diego: College-Hill Press.

Shinn, P., & Blumstein, S. (1983). Phonetic disintegration in aphasia: Acoustic analysis of spectral characteristics for place of articulation. *Brain and Language, 20*, 90–114.

Stevens, K., & Blumstein, S. (1978). Invariant cues for place of articulation in stop consonants. *Journal of the Acoustical Society of America, 64*, 1358–1368.

Sweeting, P., & Baken, R. (1982). Voice onset time in a normal-aged population. *Journal of Speech and Hearing Research, 25*, 129–134.

Trost, J., & Canter, G. (1974). Apraxia of speech in patients with Broca's aphasia: A study of phoneme production accuracy and error patterns. *Brain and Language, 1*, 63–79.

Tuller, B. (1984). On categorizing aphasic speech errors. *Neuropsychologia, 22*, 547–557.

Vowel Production in Aphasia: Towards an Account of the Consonant-Vowel Dissociation

J.H. Ryalls

A longstanding observation in aphasia is that consonant phonemes are more subject to phonemic paraphasias than are vowel phonemes. At first consideration, this fact might seem to justify less interest in vowel production after onset of aphasia, but, on the contrary, we feel that much closer investigation is warranted precisely because of this difference. In fact, this apparent difference in behavior between vowels and consonants may hold important information both about the nature of aphasia and, in a more general manner, about the process of speech production itself. This apparent difference in behavior from consonants may become one of the most important insights to be gained from investigations of vowel production in aphasia, a particular orientation that will be apparent in this chapter. Our interest thus will not only be in vowel production in aphasia itself, but especially in how it contrasts with consonant production.

The observation of a difference in the effect of aphasia on vowels when compared to consonants was first made specifically by Fry in 1959, although Alajouanine, Ombredane, and Durand (1939) had already made the suggestion of a differential phonetic disintegration for consonants versus vowels. Researchers since, who have specifically compared vowel and consonant phonemes, have continued to find this disparity in substitution errors (Shankweiler & Harris, 1966; Trost & Canter, 1974; La Pointe & Johns, 1975; Béland, 1985). Even though this observation continues to be reported, there is little in the way of a coherent hypothesis attempting to account for this difference, although there are hints scattered throughout the literature. We shall attempt to gather these shreds of evidence and to compare them in more detail—hopefully in order to arrive at a more comprehensive and systematic view of this difference between class of phoneme in aphasia.

We shall see that phonetic studies, which fractionalize phoneme production into some of its component acoustic correlates, offer the type of evidence needed to begin to account for this apparent dichotomy in phonemic production behavior Certainly the difference between consonants and vowels is not new to phonological investigations of language behavior. For example, a phonological feature that differentiates vowels and consonants in terms of phonological class is used for most accounts of linguistic patterning. In fact, the majority of phonological treatments use different sets of features for consonants than for vowels (i.e., Chomsky & Halle, 1968).

The purpose of this chapter will be to examine the differences between vowel and consonant production after aphasia at both the phonemic and the phonetic level to try and pinpoint differences that might help us to better understand the nature of this apparent dissociation. As alluded to above, the phonetic level seems to offer more pertinent information than phonemic studies in regard to this disparity, although differences in phonemic behavior will also be included in our discussion.

A primarily chronological order will be adopted in order to retain a historical notion of the development. We will start with a review of the consonant-vowel (C-V) differences at the phonemic level. Next, we will turn to phonetic studies of vowel production. This section will also serve as an overview of phonetic studies of vowel production in aphasia in general. Finally, an attempt will be made to outline possible loci for the C-V dissociation. Although such consideration will not lead us to an actual model for speech production, it is still felt that attempting, as we are here, to explain this apparent difference in speech production behavior in pathology may be stimulating for the enterprise of understanding speech behavior in general.

VOWEL PRODUCTION IN APHASIA

While it may not always be easy to maintain a clear distinction between phonemic and phonetic levels in all types of analysis, this distinction nonetheless will be used to organize the discussion. We will consider studies that rely on listeners' perception to categorize speech sounds of aphasic patients as *phonemic*; while those that use some form of instrumentation to effect acoustic measures on speech as *phonetic*.

It should also be noted here that there may be differences in the degree of this C-V dissociation according to the type of aphasic subject being considered. It is important to make sure that two different studies are both considering the same type of experimental subject. This situation seems especially sensitive in comparisons of patients with *Broca's aphasia* and those with *apraxia of speech*. For the sake of this chapter we will consider ✓ them equivalent in terms of the change in speech production. There is a similarity in the results of studies investigating each of these two patient types that justifies this conflation. But it may indeed turn out that, upon closer inspection, there are subtle differences in speech behavior that warrant their separate consideration (see Blumstein, 1981, for further discussion). In any case, for the sake of this chapter we will consider apraxia of speech as synonymous with the articulation component of Broca's aphasia, or *phonetic disintegration* (Alajouanine et al., 1939). Broca's aphasia (anterior aphasia) will, however, be distinguished from *Wernickes's aphasia* (posterior aphasia) to the extent that these two syndromes have been experimentally dissociated.

Phonemic Studies

Fry (1959) noted in his case study of the phoneme production of an aphasic patient: "The consonants accounted for rather more errors than the vowels, though the difference was not as great as might be expected; 16% of all vowels gave rise to errors, and 21% of all consonants" (p. 57). He also noted that there are no cases in which vowels have been replaced by consonants nor vice versa.

Shankweiler and Harris (1966) studied the phoneme production of a group of patients with phonetic disintegration (re: Alajouanine et al., 1939). On the basis of their results these researchers stated: "The vocalic portion of the word is produced with greater accuracy than the consonant portions." Their results led them to implicate articulatory integration as the cause for such a difference: "Thus the particular difficulty with the fricative and clusters, the frequent occurrence of errors of voicing and nasalization and the integrity of the vowels all point to a disturbance of coordinated sequencing of several articulators" (p. 288).

A form of C-V dissociation, although not specifically addressed, would be maintained in Lecours and Lhermitte's (1969) schema by consonant phonemes simply being handled by a different matrix. Although a separate matrix for vowels and consonants makes the right predictions of a difference in substitutions, it does little to explain why.

Trost and Canter (1974) concluded in a similar vein to that of Shankweiler and Harris, on the basis of their study of Broca's aphasics with apraxia of speech: "Vowels were produced more accurately than are singleton consonants" (p.77). The authors make a further observation: "The nature of the majority of errors made on vowels suggested that vowels were misarticulated in relation to articulatory difficulty on contiguous consonants; that is, difficulty in articulating the CV or VC transition (and/or in selecting the consonant phoneme(s) seemed to cause the vowel nucleus to become distorted. There were no instances in which a vowel error constituted the only error in production of a monosyllabic word" (p. 70).

Such a statement seems to predict that aphasic patients will only make errors on vowel phonemes due to "spreading" of the articulatory difficulty from the consonant phonemes. Studies of coarticulation in aphasia should help us to assess this issue more directly (See Ziegler & von Cramon (1985, 1986) as well as Katz & Tuller in Chapters 11 and 12.)

LaPointe and Johns (1975) have also made very similar conclusions about a C-V dissociation in the speech of Broca's aphasics with apraxia of speech: "Consonants were more susceptible to error than were vowels" (p. 259).

Even though one regularly meets with the observation in the literature that consonant phonemes give rise to many more substitutions than do vowel phonemes, it must be mentioned that this observation is not universal. For example, Lebrun et al., (1973) present results of two case studies of patients with anarthria, one of whom presented with more vowel than consonant substitutions. "Of a theoretical total of 572 vowels, Joseph made 35 mistakes, i.e. 6.1%; of a total of 739 consonants, he made 40 mistakes, i.e. 5.4%. The corresponding percentages for our second patient are 2.6% and 13.7%. Thus only our second case conforms to the widely-held view that in anarthria vowel production is on the whole less disturbed than consonantal production" (p. 35).

Keller (1975) also noted that the subjects used in his study responded to more opportunities for vowel substitutions than one would expect from the literature. In any case, these two exceptions notwithstanding, it is still the majority of phonological analyses of speech after left cortical damage (i.e., any type of aphasia) that have found a C-V disparity.

In a very recent phonological study of substitutions completed by Béland (1985), using a *tridimensional approach*, which allows one to account for phonological aspects of syllabicity, a similar C-V dissociation was noted for different aphasic syndromes. (For motivation of phonological status of the syllable the reader is referred to Selkirk, 1982.) The author notes: "We see first of all that for the majority of aphasic and normal groups, the number of simple consonantal substitutions is greater than the number of simple vowel substitutions in repetition. . . These results are in agreement with numerous studies which have reported a greater number of consonantal than vocalic substitutions. . . The strong position that the vowel occupies in the syllable is certainly not unrelated to this fact" (p. 96).

By "strong position" Béland was referring to the privileged role that vowel positions play in syllabification. In phonological accounts that use the syllable as a structural unit, one begins to suspect that vowel positions may indeed provide more basic structural information than are given by consonant positions. Furthermore, she noted: "Upon inspection, it is revealed that 72.5% (427) of vowel substitutions made by aphasics depend on vowels in un-accented positions; compared to 27.5% (162) of the substitutions for accented vowels, that is belonging to the last syllable of the word."[1]

Béland's results, especially vis-a-vis accented versus unaccented syllables, suggest a possible prosodic factor in the C-V dissociation. For example, consonants cannot carry stress, and it is those vowels which also are unaccented that are more likely to result in substitutions. Such a difference seems rather related to the stress-saliency hypothesis proposed by Goodglass, Fodor, and Schulhoff (1967) to account for words that are most likely to be retained by agrammatic patients. This issue will be considered in greater detail in the section on possible explanations for the C-V dissociation. However, changes are noted in syllabic amplitude in aphasic speech revealed by Kent and Rosenbek (1983), discussed in the section on amplitude in the following section on instrumental analyses. A discussion of phonetic or instrumental studies of vowel production in aphasia follows.

Phonetic Studies

The first instrumental analysis of aphasic speech is, to the author's knowledge that of Alajouanine and colleagues in 1939. Although limited to Rousselot cylinders, a kind of prototype oscillograph that records speech vibrations onto a revolving cylinder, these researchers were able to instrumentally document some of the acoustic characteristics of the syndrome that they baptized *phonetic disintegration*. The Rousselot cylinder was useful for measuring timing characteristics, although fundamental frequency could also probably be measured by counting the number of periods per some unit of time. However, such an instrument could not be used to execute a spectral analysis, which would have to wait for the advent of the sound spectrograph.

Alajouanine and colleagues (1939) also seem to have developed the first explanatory hypothesis for a differentiation of consonant and vowel articulation in aphasia. This hypothesis has probably gone somewhat unnoticed because these same authors do not really document the greater number of phonemic substitutions for consonants in aphasia. Nonetheless the following statement in the summary section of their monograph on phonetic disintegration is surprisingly explicit in regard to this dissociation: "The articulatory movements offer a syn-kinetic character, and a phoneme will have much more of a chance of being emitted if its pronunciation is compatible with a more global, less differentiated action of the phonatory organs. This is the case in the oral vowels for which the phases

---

[1]Word-accent in French is always on the last syllable of the word; unlike English where it changes, often according to the phonological form of the word. Thus stress has no lexical status in French, whereas it does in English.)

of tension and release have much less importance than for the consonants" (p. 119).

From this point on, for the sake of clarity, the dicussion will be divided by the individual acoustic correlates under consideration, starting with duration.

Duration

Alajouanine and colleagues (1939) note the prolongation of the vowel traces produced by their aphasic patients in comparison to those of their normal speakers. However, there were no group comparisons nor were statistics used to test the significance of this effect. Since variability seems to be a cardinal feature of aphasic speech, it is important to know if the lengthening effect is significant, in spite of increased variability.

Shankweiler, Harris, and Taylor (1968) described longer vowels as one of the features of phonetic disintegration revealed by their EMG study: "vowels were prolonged and variable in length" (p. 8). (Note that this variability turns out to be an important descriptive factor in aphasia, and may even turn out to be the most consistent feature revealed by instrumental analyses of aphasic speech.) The study allowed the authors to attempt to define phonetic disintegration with more precision: "All the findings point to a disturbance of coordinated sequencing of several articulators" (p. 6).

Lebrun et al. (1973) noted of their anarthric patient: "Joseph's articulation is slower than that of normal speakers. . . Oscillographic investigation reveals that this longer time is not due to blocks. Phonemes simply take longer, i.e., the articulation is slower" (p. 127). This finding was confirmed more recently for a group of motor (Broca's) aphasics in which lengthening was found at the level of the sentence, the word, and the vowel phoneme (Ryalls, 1981). Thus the lengthening was not simply due to the insertion of pauses.

In a spectrographic analysis Kent and Rosenbek (1982) also found: "The apractic speech patterns that we observed were reduced in rate relative to normal speech. The slowing of rate took two major forms: articulatory prolongation and syllable segregation" (pp. 264–265). Likewise were their results, published in 1983: "All seven apraxic subjects had slow speaking rate compared to the seven normally speaking controls" (p. 233). However, the authors also found that the magnitude of the lengthening effect was increased as the length of the utterance increased: "Thus, vowel lengthening for the apraxic speakers increased as syllabic length of utterance increased" (p. 234–235). The author will return to this point in summarizing the published instrumental results on vowel production in aphasia.

Collins, Rosenbek, and Wertz (1983) compared apraxic and normal speakers' phonemic productions and concluded: "Our results revealed that both groups reduced the vowel duration as words increased in length. Word and vowel durations for apraxia of speech patients, however, were often significantly larger than those for normal speakers" (p. 224).

Gandour and Dardarananda (1984) also studied vowel duration in a group of Thai brain-damaged speakers and compared them to normal native speakers. These authors wished to see if aphasic speakers were still capable of maintaining the long–short phonological contrast in Thai. They found that their patients retained the phonological length distinction, and, in fact, there was no significant overall lengthening effect. They further noted: "Of the brain-damaged subjects, only the dysarthric patient exhibits average duration values which are considerably longer than normal for both vowel length categories. . . The duration ratios for all the brain-damaged patients fall within or just outside the range for the normal group" (p. 215). On the basis of their results, these authors summarized: "The data from the language tests indicate that both of our Broca's aphasics experienced considerable difficulty in the production of articulatory sequences. However, their articulatory difficulties do not apparently extend to the timing control of vowel duration in monosyllabic words" (p.217).

It should be noted here that the target words of all of the studies mentioned above that have found longer durations for apraxic and aphasic speakers are all polysyllabic. There are two other studies of vowel duration that used monosyllabic stimuli (CVC words) for target productions. These are Duffy and Gawle (1984) and Ryalls (1984). Neither found significant lengthening for the apraxic or anterior aphasics (respectively).

Ryalls (1986) found the variability in vowel duration productions (from repetition to repetition) to be significantly greater than normal in the group of anterior (Broca's) aphasics. In this study, although the aphasic patients' durations were always numerically larger than those for the normal subjects, they were not significantly longer. In fact it was the posterior aphasics who presented the largest overall average duration.

In summary, it seems that aphasic patients are generally longer in vowel production than normal subjects, but this effect only seems to reach statistical significance when the target word is polysyllabic. Thus vowels were longer (significantly when statistics were used) in all studies that compared polysyllabic words in aphasics to polysyllabic words in normal controls. Two studies that used CVC stimuli did not find a significant lengthening effect. This issue should be investigated in greater detail, but so far the results seem to suggest that the degree of disintegration (at least as revealed by duration measures) may be dependent upon the length of the utterance unit to be programmed.

Kent and Rosenbek (1983) have interpreted the increasing difficulty factor to be due to one of two factors: "The lengthening of segments and the errors in the control of relative segment duration could be ascribed either to errors at a high level of motor programming or to unreliable reafferent information concerning the timing of movements" (p. 245). In Kent and Rosenbek's interpretation unreliable reafferent information might cause a patient to prolong articulation "possibly in an attempt to gather the required sensory information by which the antecedent motor program can be evaluated" (p. 246).

However, the issue of syllabic complexity must also be considered—especially in terms of lexical accent. That is, a CVC word has a perfectly predictable stress pattern: The single syllabic nuclei present will receive the accent. A longer word presents a more complex accentuation, as there are more potential positions for stress placement. Since duration interacts with stress placement, this aspect of increasing phonological complexity in conjunction with longer words should not be ignored in studies of vowel duration in aphasia.

Amplitude

Although there are only two instrumental studies that have addressed vowel amplitude in aphasic speech production, the results are interesting enough to merit a rather detailed discussion. Let us note, however, that studies of amplitude are extremely limited at the present time.

The first instrumental study of amplitude measures is the previously cited case study of anarthria by Lebrun et al. (1973). The authors noted: "The amplitude of most vowels is much greater than that of adjacent consonants, so that, in contradistinction to ordinary speech (Lebrun, 1966), practically each syllable is marked by a 'peak of prominence' to use Jones' phrase (Jones, 1960, p. 55, cited in Lebrun, 1966). These peaks tend to be equally spaced, i.e. most syllables are isochronous" (p. 127).

This result is reminiscent of one of Alajouanine et al.'s (1939) elements of the syndrome of phonetic disintegration in aphasia, namely: "When the patient is capable of polysyllabic utterances, the syllables are detached, uttered slowly and difficultly, one after the other, the tonic accent has disappeared, the 'melody of language' is lost" (p. 121).

In 1983, Kent and Rosenbek published their comprehensive acoustic study: "Acoustic patterns of apraxia of speech." This work offers the most extensive comparison of suprasegmental and segmental aspects of pathological speech production to date. Kent and Rosenbek's study was especially pertinent in its results for amplitude. These authors found that the major difference was that apraxic subjects showed less variation in relative peak intensity across syllables. . . The results conform to the expectation that the apraxic speakers would display a flattening of the intensity envelope across a syllabic sequence" (p. 237).

This difference in relative intensity differentiation for two sentences produced by an apraxic group and a normal control group was also tested statistically and found to be significant (p. 26). Kent and Rosenbek continue: "The mean relative reduction was consistently smaller for the apraxic speakers than for the normal speakers. In practical terms, this means that normally reduced syllables, especially function words like 'the,' 'in,' 'on,' and 'was,' are relatively more intense in apraxic speech than in normal speech" (p. 237).

This result is especially interesting in light of the known tendency for agrammatic Broca's aphasics to drop just these speech elements in their speech. In fact, Goodglass and colleagues (1967) have suggested that these elements drop out because of their lack of prominence. The fact that when they are indeed retained, they are produced with greater acoustic prominence than normal is an intriguing result and one that demands greater attention. But further consideration of the relationship between phonetic realization and agrammatic aspects of aphasic speech is beyond the scope of this chapter. Suffice it to note that aphasic patients with speech production problems seem to significantly reduce the normal acoustic differences in syllabic prominence.

Fundamental Frequency

Very few studies have specifically investigated the realization of the fundamental frequency at the segmental level. Of course the *timing* of voicing is well studied in the VOT literature (See Blumstein & Baum, Chapter 1), but the *frequency* of the fundamental is rarely measured in vowel production, probably because it is not related to a linguistic contrast. Most studies of fundamental frequency are concerned with its modulation at the level of sentence production where it is referred to as *intonation*. (The reader is referred to Cooper & Klouda in Chapter 4). In any case, two studies have effected such measures. Kent and Rosenbek (1983) note that even after apraxic speaker's *fundamental frequency* (F_O) values were normalized for difference in utterance duration and mean values, there was a large degree of interspeaker variability. However, no differences in mean F_O of apraxic versus normal speakers were noted.

In a 1984 study by Ryalls, the F_O was measured at the midpoint of each 45 vowel productions produced by a group of 5 anterior and 7 posterior aphasics and compared them statistically to those for 7 normal speakers. The anterior aphasics were significantly higher in overall F_O than the normals speakers but not significantly different than posterior aphasics. Posterior aphasics were not significantly higher than normal subjects. In any case, it was suggested that the higher average vocal frequency of Broca's aphasics could be due to their higher psychological stress in read speech production (Ryalls, 1984), but more research should be addressed to this possible effect.

An evaluation of variability of F_O measures at the midpoint of the vowel productions was also conducted. This analysis revealed that anterior aphasics produced significantly greater variability in vowel durations than did the normal subjects (Ryalls, 1984). We shall see that this increased variability in acoustic realization of speech by anterior aphasics (Broca's aphasics, verbal apraxics) seems to be a consistent feature of acoustic analyses, no matter what the correlate being measured (*duration*: Shankweiler et al., 1968; Ryalls, 1984; *formant frequency patterning*: Keller, 1975; Ryalls, 1981; 1986; *fundamental frequency*: Kent and Rosenbek, 1982; Ryalls, 1984; *EMG measures*: Shankweiler et al., 1968; *velum lowering*: Itoh, Sasanuma, & Ushijima, 1982; *VOT*: Blumstein et al., 1980).

Formant Frequency Targeting

The first spectral study of vowel production in aphasia proper, is that of Keller (1975). Keller found that his aphasic speakers produced more variability in formant frequencies than did normal subjects. This change was in the opposite direction from that of dysarthic speakers (Tikofsky, 1968). It suggests that the aphasic speakers do not have a limitation of tongue mobility, and in fact that their productions are more variable than those of normal speakers. However, Keller also found that there were differences in mean formant values for the aphasic subjects compared to the normal speakers. That is: "The aphasic vowel configurations appear to be somewhat flattened along the F1 axis, in comparison to the normal configuration. With the exception of [ə], aphasic vowels have a higher F1 than normal vowels." Keller interpreted these results in terms of wider vocal tract configurations on the part of the aphasic speakers.

Keller's results for greater formant variability were essentially replicated with a group of exclusively anterior aphasics in another spectrographic study (Ryalls, 1981). Also there were a few instances in which one or the other of the formant frequencies were significantly different for the aphasic patients than for the normal subjects However no consistent direction was observed for these changes.

Kent and Rosenbek (1983) have also contributed a spectrographic analysis of vowel production in apraxia of speech as part of their larger study. They revealed some individual abnormalities in the patient's vowel production. But their subjects "have a satisfactory overall range of F1–F2 values for the English vowel system. However, some individual productions were extremely deviant in F1-F2 pattern" (p. 242).

A computer-implemented acoustic analysis of vowel production in aphasia, explicity contrasting anterior and posterior aphasics, was recently completed (Ryalls, 1986). The study also included a comparison of intra-individual variability. Acoustic vowel plots for three of the nine vowels from that study are presented in Figures 2-1, 2-2, and 2-3. Each figure plots vowel productions with F1 on the verticle axis and F2 of the horizontal axis. The top plot (N)is for the normal subjects (7 subjects × 5 repetitions); the middle plot (A) is for the anterior aphasics (5 subjects × 5 repetitions)

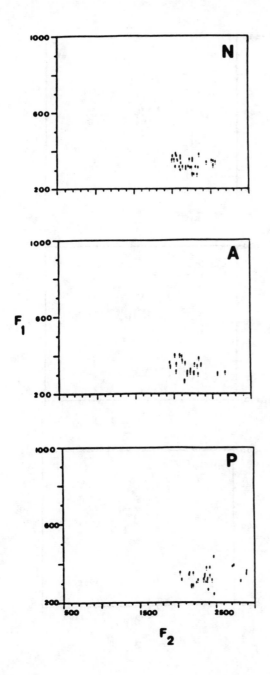

FIGURE 2-1. Acoustic plots of five 'heed' vowels produced by seven Normal speakers (N), five Anterior aphasics (A) and seven Posterior aphasics (P).

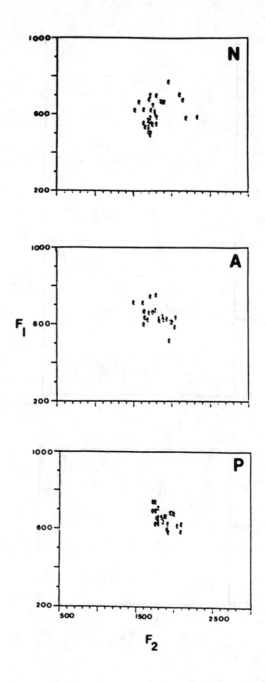

FIGURE 2-2. Acoustic plots of five 'had' vowels produced by seven Normal speakers (N), five Anterior aphasics (A), and seven Posterior aphasics (P).

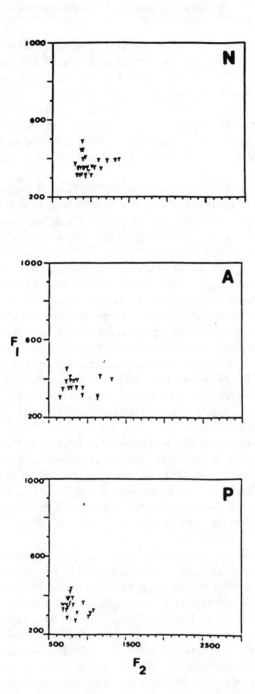

FIGURE 2-3. Acoustic plots of five 'who'd' vowels produced by seven Normal speakers (N), five Anterior aphasics (A), and seven Posterior aphasics (P).

and the bottom plot (P) is for the posterior aphasics (7 subjects × 5 repetitions). Figure 2-1 is for the vowel from *heed*, Figure 2-2 the vowel from *had* and Figure 2-3 the vowel from *who'd*. Looking at these figures, no systematic differences are discernable, either in the placement of vowel productions or in the spread of the vowels in the acoustic space. Of course in these figures the repetitions for a particular subject cannot be distinguished from those of other subjects, but a statistical analysis revealed no difference from normal subjects in average formant values for either aphasic group.

Even though a normalization procedure was also effected on the formant values to compensate for possible difference in vocal tract length among the subjects, and although normal subjects were taken from the same dialect area, no significant differences between groups were found for average formant frequency means (Ryalls, 1986). This result suggests that the vowel targets towards which aphasic patients are aiming their productions are essentially the same as those for normal subjects.

However, another statistical analysis performed on the standard deviations of five repetitions of the same target vowel revealed that both types of aphasic patients were significantly less accurate in keeping on target from production to production. Since phonemic substitutions were not included in the acoustic analyses, these results suggest that there is a substantial degree of articulatory "noise" in vowel productions on the part of aphasic patients, which is not apparent in simple ear-analysis. This result points out the degree to which simple transcriptions of speech production in aphasia may be limited.

The study did not find any significant differences in the formant frequency means, and the result is different in this particular respect from Keller (1975) and Ryalls (1981). In any case, additional studies will be required to replicate the results outlined above. What is a point of agreement is that aphasic patients are more variable in their formant frequency productions of vowels, both as a group (Keller, 1975; Ryalls, 1981) and as individuals (Ryalls, 1986).

Sussman and colleagues (1986) have recently completed an investigation of Broca's aphasics' vowel production under bite-block constraint. The authors found acoustic evidence that Broca's aphasics are less able to compensate restricted articulation. Furthermore, since it was particularly those patients with damage to Brodman's area 44 who were implicated, these authors assign a special role to this area in articulatory compensation. In light of the phonetic outputting differences found in Wernicke (posterior) aphasics as well in Ryalls (1986), however, it seems important to test posterior aphasics as well, before a privileged role for compensation can be assigned to area 44.

Summary

From the author's review of phonemic studies, it has been seen that most studies have found vowels to be more resistant to phonemic substitution than are consonants. This finding seems to be corroborated by studies at the phonetic level, but a direct comparison is rather preliminary at this stage; i.e., there is a problem in comparing degree of phonetic disintegration across acoustic dimensions: for example, how does one compare formant frequency patterning to voice-onset time (VOT) production? There is also the problem that the comparison of vowels and consonants at the phonetic level has not been made for the same subject's speech production. Also, for the instrumental studies that will be compared here, measures of vowel formant patterning eliminated phonemic substitutions before acoustic measures were effected (Ryalls, 1986), whereas acoustic measures were effected on the whole corpus for consonants (Blumstein et al., 1980; Shinn & Blumstein, 1983).

In spite of these apparent problems, the author feels that a comparison between phonetic outputting for vowels and consonants can be made. It does not seem to be the case that the in-between phonemic category productions for VOT of consonants (especially for Broca or anterior aphasics) (Blumstein et al. 1980) is seen in vowel production of formant frequencies (Ryalls, 1986). Furthermore, when a more static acoustic feature such as place of articulation for consonants is considered (Shinn & Blumstein, 1983), the same degree of disintegration is not seen. We thus suspect that it is the fine degree of *temporal integration* of articulators that is required for proper realization of VOT that does not seem to be necessary for either place of articulation or for formant frequency production that seems especially implicated in aphasia (especially Broca's aphasia). Recall that both Alajouanine et al. (1939) and Shankweiler et al. (1966, 1968) have implicated lack of integration of articulators as a general factor resulting in phonetic disintegration in aphasia.

Note also that while there seems to be a significant difference in the degree of phonetic disintegration of consonants for VOT between anterior (Broca) and posterior (Wernicke) aphasias (Blumstein et al., 1980), such a difference does not seem to be maintained in formant frequency targeting of vowels (Ryalls, 1986).

THE CONSONANT-VOWEL DISSOCIATION

Let us take this differential disintegration of consonants and vowels as a working hypothesis for aphasia. More experimentation is surely in order, but we believe that there is enough evidence of a difference between vowel and consonant production in aphasia to warrent consideration of possible explanations for this apparent dissociation. As mentioned, temporal integration of articulators seems to be one of the most relevant differences between consonant and vowel production; but there are several other possible factors that could well be implicated. The following outlines some of the possible factors possibly entering into the consonant vowel dissociation. These factors can only be considered in a rather superficial manner here, as there is not enough evidence to decide between possible causes. Consideration of these possible causes for a difference between vowels and consonants is also worthwhile in that this dissociation seems a part of the normal speech system and not something that aphasia introduces. In other words, studies of aphasia seem to reveal an apparently natural dissociation inherent in human speech. Although aphasia may indeed exaggerate this dissociation, we consider the difference to be an integral part of the normal system.

In this final section, some of the aspects of normal speech perception and production that might help understanding this apparent dissociation of vowels and consonants can be briefly considered. First, some aspects of speech perception will be considered. Bond (1981) has shown that vowel distortion provoked poorer comprehension in listeners of elliptic speech than other consonant distortions. This result may suggest that the relative preservation of vowel production is integral to retaining comprehension of aphasic speech.

One of the most significant insights into the nature of speech perception which highlighted its apparently "special" perceptual status was that of its categorical nature (Liberman et al., 1967). That is, on the one hand, there were rather large physical differences on a continuum within a phoneme category that were essentially ignored by listeners, while, on the other, listeners were quite sensitive to rather small physical differences in a continuum at the border between two categories (see Repp, 1983, for a review). At least in the early categorical perception experiments, vowels did not demonstrate the same boundary discrimination peaks of catgorical perception as found with consonant stimuli (Fry, et al., 1962). Although later studies have indeed found evidence for boundary peaks (Fujisaki & Kawashima, 1969; 1970; Pisoni, 1971), there is still an apparent difference in the degree to which consonants are categorically perceived in comparison to vowels.

The results of categorical perception in regard to phoneme class are also reflected in dichotic listening studies. While stop consonants gave rather consistent right ear advantages (REA's)—presumably reflecting the superior capacity of the left hemisphere for processing such speech stimuli—vowels did not (Shankweiler & Studdert-Kennedy, 1966; 1967; Studdert-Kennedy & Shankweiler, 1970). This contrasting result was explained by appealing to the degree of *encodedness*. That is, consonants have to undergo more extensive restructuring of the acoustic signal (Liberman, 1974).

Schwartz and Tallal (1980) have claimed that it is the difference in the rate of acoustic change between consonants and vowels which accounts for consonants being more laterally perceived and vowels not giving clear ear effects. However Dwyer, Blumstein, and Ryalls (1982) have challenged this claim with results that show that it is not simply the difference in duration, but also the nature of the acoustic cue that affects the degree of lateralization. Such considerations lead us to consider differences in how consonants and vowels are produced.

One of the most extensive investigations of speech production behavior to date also led to postulation of a "functional division of articulatory activity into two classes" (Perkell, 1969). Perkell stated:

> Many parts of the vocal tract play a role in the production of both vowels and consonants, but in general the same organs seem to behave differently under the influence of the two different classes. Consonant articulations by the tongue and lips are generally observed to be faster and more geometrically complex, and they require more precision in timing than vowel articulations. . . .The general differences in velocity, complexity, precision of movement and in anatomy suggest that different types of muscles are generally responsible for C and V production. It is probable that articulation of vowels is accomplished principally by the slower extrinsic tongue musculature which controls tongue position. On the other hand, consonant articulation requires the addition of more precise more complex and faster function of the smaller intrinsic tongue musculature. (p. 61)

A similar functional division of phoneme classes was already argued for by Ohman (1966; 1967). More recently, Fowler and colleagues (1980) have also considered reasons for such a functional division as follows: "they (vowels) are *separate* from consonants (and hence their serial ordering with respect to consonants can be detected by a perceivor) because the organizational invariants for vowels perpetrate a different *kind* of articulatory and acoustic event than those for consonants" (p. 413).

Considering the acoustic nature of vowels versus consonants, it can also be suggested that vowels are more redundant than are consonants, and therefore more resistant to noise. Since the vowel portion of the acoustic waveform is already a much more regular repeating pattern, it can be readily predicted to be much more resistant to random fluctuations than is a consonantal portion.

Vowels have acoustic information relevant to their perception *distributed* rather diffusely throughout their duration; while in consonants the relevant acoustic information seems much more *discrete*, and localized at the onset. (See also Stevens & Blumstein, 1978, and Blumstein &

Stevens, 1979, for discussion of the abrupt nature of consonant perception). This difference is often referred to as *abrupt* versus *steady-state*.

It is interesting to consider in our comparison of vowels and consonants that vowels (or at least vocoid-like productions) seem to be acquired earlier by children than do consonant phonemes (Locke, 1983). In phonological treatments that appeal to syllabic structure, information about vowel positions is more basic than information about consonantal positions, given the privileged role of the vowel in determining syllabification.

Jonathan Kaye (personal communication) is developing a phonological theory of "charm and government" in collaboration with colleagues, wherein the more basic role of the vowel class of phoneme would be given a formalization. That is, in such a theory, consonant phonemes are derived from underlying vowels. In fact such a model would make the more basic nature of vowels rather explicit. (The reader is referred to Kaye, Lowenstamm, & Vergnaud (1985) for the basic features of the model.) Note that such a treatment may also imply that vowels are perhaps more "primordial" or "older" in terms of evolving phonological systems. This proposal that vowels are more basic may find an interpretation in terms of 'microgeny' in which the steps of cognition (in this case, the developing speech act) follow similar steps as those of ontogeny and phylogeny (Brown, 1977). It would come as no surprise to such a theoretical formulation that children acquire vowel sounds earlier, and that one finds vowel-like sounds further down the phylogenetic scale than man. But it must be noted that we have no clear understanding in this area.

In summary, the picture that seems to be emerging from comparison of consonant and vowel behavior in the language system is that vowels are somehow more basic or 'prime' and consequently (and perhaps fortuitously) more resistant to phonetic disintegration in aphasia. Vowel positions seem to be more integral to the timing and prosodic envelope of a particular utterance. We can speculate further that it was the development of the highly precise and automated articulation found in stop consonants that allowed for the extremely fast (i.e. encoded) transmission rates found in human speech. The faster and more integrated articulation found in stop consonants also seem more dependent upon a specialized mechanism that seems to be found (at least in most right handers) in the anterior portion (Broca's area) of the left hemisphere of the human brain. Thus it is the most highly integrated components of human speech that seem most susceptible to neurological damage to this area.

This seems to be the formulation neccessary to explain the fact that aphasia affects consonant production to a greater degree than that of vowels and furthermore that it is especially damage to the anterior portion, or Broca's area, of the left hemisphere that results in this partially selective deficit of consonants.

We see that the disintegration of the language system brought about by aphasia is still ordered by the same principles that govern intact function.

By studying this disintegration we stand to gather greater insights into the functioning of the normal system. One sees in this intact organization just how highly structured and resistant to disorganization the intact language system is. It survives even an assault as severe as aphasia largely, but not entirely, intact. Less severe assaults such as bite-block (Lindblom, Lubker, & Gay, 1979) and nerve-block (Bordon, 1978) seem to leave the normal system's functioning almost entirely unaffected. Since aphasia does indeed succeed in partially destructuring normal speech production, it holds a rich potential in revealing the organization of the system.

REFERENCES

Alajouanine, T., Ombredane, A., & Durand, M. (1939). *Le syndrome de désintegration phonétique dans l'aphasie.* Paris: Masson et Cie.

Béland, R. (1985). Constraintes syllabiques sur les erreurs phonologiques dans l'aphasie (unpublished Ph.D. dissertation, Université de Montréal).

Blumstein, S. (1981). Phonological aspects of aphasia. In M.T. Sarno (Ed.), *Acquired aphasia.* New York: Academic Press.

Blumstein, S., & Stevens, K. (1979). Acoustic invariance in speech production: Evidence from measurements of the spectral characteristics of stop consonants. *Journal of the Acoustical Society of America, 66*(4): 1001–1017.

Blumstein, S., Cooper, W., Goodglass, H., Statlender, S., & Gottlieb, J. (1980). Production deficits in aphasia: A voice-onset-time analysis. *Brain and Language, 9,* 153–170.

Bond, Z. (1981). Listening to elliptic speech: Pay attention to stressed vowels. *Journal of Phonetics, 9,* 89–96.

Bordon, G. (1979). An interpretation of research on feedback interruption in speech. *Brain and Language, 7,* 307–319.

Brown, J. (1977) *Mind, brain and consciousness: The neuropsychology of cognition.* New York: Academic Press.

Chomsky, N., & Halle, M. (1968). *The sound pattern of English.* New York: Harper and Row.

Collins, M., Rosenbek, J., & Wertz, R. (1983). Spectrographic analysis of vowel and word duration in apraxia of speech. *Journal of Speech and Hearing Research, 26,* 224–230.

Duffy, J., & Gawle, C. (1984). Apraxic speaker's vowel duration in consonant-vowel-consonant syllables. In J. Rosenbek, M. McNeil, & A. Aronson (Eds.), *Apraxia of speech: Physiology, acoustics, linguistics, management.* San Diego: College Hill Press.

Dwyer, J., Blumstein, S., & Ryalls, J. (1982). The role of duration and rapid temporal processing on the lateral perception of consonants and vowels. *Brain and Language, 17,* 272–286.

Fowler, C., Rubin, P., Remez, R., & Turvey, M. (1980). Implications for speech production of a general theory of action. In B. Butterworth (Ed.), *Language production volume one: Speech and talk.* London: Academic Press.

Fry, D. (1959). Phonemic substitutions in an aphasic patient. *Language and Speech, 2,* 52–61.

Fry, D., Abramson, A., Eimas, P., & Liberman, A. (1962). The identification and discrimination of synthetic speech sounds. *Language and Speech, 5,* 171–189.

Fujisaki, H., & Kawashima, T. (1969). On the modes and mechanisms of speech perception. *Annual Report of the Engineering Research Institute, Faculty of Engineering, University of Tokyo, 28,* 67–73.

Fujisaki , H., & Kawashima, T. (1970). Some experiments on speech perception and a model for the perceptual mechanisms. *Annual Report of the Engineering Research Institute, Faculty of Engineering, University of Tokyo, 29,* 207–214.

Gandour, J., & Dardarananda, R. (1984). Prosodic disturbance in aphasia: Vowel length in Thai. *Brain and Language, 23,* 206–224.

Goodglass, H., Fodor, I.,& Schulhoff, C. (1967). Prosodic factors in grammar—evidence from aphasia. *Journal of Speech and Hearing Research, 10,* 5–20.

Itoh, M., Sasanuma, S., & Ushijima, T. (1979). Velar movements during speech in a patient with apraxia of speech. *Brain and Language, 7,* 227–239.

Kaye, J., Lowenstamm, J., & Vergnaud, J.-R. (1985). The internal stucture of phonological elements: A theory of charm and government. *Phonology Yearbook, 2,* 305–328.

Keller, E. (1975). Vowel errors in aphasia. (Unpublished Ph.D. dissertation, University of Toronto).

Kent, R., & Rosenbek, J. (1982). Prosodic disturbance and neurologic lesion. *Brain and Language, 15,* 259–291.

Kent, R., & Rosenbek, J. (1983). Acoustic patterns of apraxia of speech. *Journal of Speech and Hearing Research, 26,* 231–249.

LaPointe, L., & Johns, D. (1975). Some phonemic characteristics in apraxia of speech. *Journal of Communication Disorders, 8,* 259–269.

Lebrun, Y., Buyssens, E., & Henneaux, J. (1973). Phonetic aspects of anarthria. *Cortex, 9,* 126–135.

Lecours, A.R., & Lhermitte, F. Phonemic paraphasias: Linguistic structures and tentative hypotheses. *Cortex 5,* 193–338.

Liberman, A. (1974). The specialization of the language hemisphere. In F. Schmitt & F. Worden (Eds.), *The neurosciences third study program.* Cambridge, MA: M.I.T. Press.

Liberman, A., Cooper, F., Shankweiler, D., & Studdert-Kennedy, M. (1967). Perception of the speech code. *Psychological Review, 74,* 431–461.

Lindblom, B., Lubker, J., & Gay, T. (1979). Formant frequencies of some fixed-mandible vowels and a model of speech motor programming by predictive simulation. *Journal of Phonetics, 7,* 147–161.

Locke, J. (1983). *Phonological acquisition and change.* New York: Academic Press.

MacNeilage, P., Studdert-Kennedy, M., & Lindblom, B. (1985). Planning and Production of speech: An overview. In J. Lanter (Ed.), *Proceedings of the Conference on Planning and Production of Speech by Normally Hearing and Deaf People.* (ASHA Reports No. 15) St. Louis, MO: ASHA.

Ohman, S. (1966). Coarticulation in VCV utterances: Spectrographic measurements. *Journal of the Acoustical Society of America, 39,* 151–168.

Ohman, S. (1967). Numerical model of coarticulation. *Journal of the Acoustical Society of America, 41,* 310–320.

Perkell, J. (1969). *Physiology of speech production: Results and implication of a quantitative cineradiographic study.* Research monograph No. 53. Cambridge, MA: MIT Press.

Pisoni, D. (1971). On the nature of categorical perception of speech sounds (Unpublished Ph.D. dissertation, The University of Michigan).

Repp, B. (1983). Categorical preception: Issues, methods, findings. In N. Lass (Ed.) *Speech and language: Advances in basic research and practice.* New York: Academic Press.

Ryalls, J. (1981). Motor aphasia: Acoustic correlates of phonetic disintegration in vowels. *Neuropsychologia 19,* 365–374.

Ryalls, J. (1984). Some acoustic correlates of F_O of CVC utterances in aphasia. *Phonetica, 41,* 103–111.

Ryalls, J. (1986). A study of vowel production in aphasia. *Brain and Language,* 29, 48–67.

Schwartz, J., & Tallal, P. (1980). Rate of acoustic change may underlie hemispheric specialization for speech perception. *Science, 207,* 1380–1381.

Selkirk, E. (1982). The syllable. In H. van der Hulst & N. Smith (Eds.), *The structure of phonological representations* (Part II), Dordrecht: Foris Publications.

Shankweiler, D., & Harris, K. (1966). An experimental approach to the problem of articulation in aphasia. *Cortex, 2,* 277–292.

Shankweiler, D., Harris, K., & Taylor, M. (1968). Electromyographic studies of articulation in aphasia. *Archives of Physical Medicine and Rehabilitation, 49,* 1–8.

Shankweiler, D., and Studdert-Kennedy, M. (1966). Lateral differences in perception of dichotically presented CV syllables and steady-state vowels. *Journal of the Acoustical Society of America, 39,* 1256.

Shankweiler, D., & Studdert-Kennedy, M. (1967). Identification of consonants and vowels presented to right and left ears. *Quarterly Journal of Experimental Psychology, 19,* 59–63.

Shinn, P., & Blumstein, S. (1983). Phonetic disintegration in aphasia: Acoustic analysis of spectral characteristics for place of articulation. *Brain and Language,* 20, 90–114.

Stevens, K., & Blumstein, S. (1978). Invariant cues for place of articulation in stop consonants. *Journal of the Acoustical Society of America, 64,* 1358–1368.

Studdert-Kennedy, M., & Shankweiler, D. (1970). Hemispheric specialization for speech perception. *Journal of the Acoustical Society of America, 48,* 579–594.

Sussman, H., Marquardt, T., Hutchinson, J., & MacNeilage, P. (1986). Compensatory articulation in Broca's aphasia. *Brain and Language, 27,* 56–74.

Tikofsky, R. (1965). *Phonetic characteristics of dysarthria.* Ann Arbor: Office of Research Administration, The University of Michigan.

Trost, J., & Canter, G. (1974). Apraxia of speech in patients with Broca's aphasia: A study of phoneme production accuracy and error patterns. *Brain and Language,* 1, 63–79.

Ziegler, W., & von Cramon, D. (1985). Anticipatory coarticulation in a patient with apraxia of speech. *Brain and Language, 26,* 117–130.

Ziegler, W., & von Cramon, D. (1986). Disturbed coarticulation in apraxia of speech: Acoustic evidence. *Brain and Language, 29,* 34–47.

C H A P T E R 3

Tone Production in Aphasia

Jack Gandour

Prosodic features of speech refer to variations in three acoustical properties of the speech waveform: duration, amplitude, and fundamental frequency (F_O). The principal linguistic correlates of these attributes include stress, intonation, tone, length, and rhythm. Because these acoustical properties systematically correspond to features of linguistic structure, we can acquire knowledge about the structure and processing of language by measuring these acoustical properties of the speech wave (e.g., Cooper & Sorensen, 1981). In recent years, speech prosody has become an increasingly useful medium for studying the role of the left and right hemispheres in the control of these acoustical properties in both linguistic and emotional domains, and for studying language representation and processing in different types of aphasia. Several studies of the production of speech prosody in brain-damaged patients have been conducted with native speakers of English (e.g., Weintraub et al., 1981; Danly & Shapiro, 1982; Danly et al., 1983; Kent and Rosenbek, 1983; Shapiro and Danly, 1985; Cooper et al., 1984). In contrast, very little information is available on speech prosody in brain-damaged patients who are native speakers of a *tone language*.

By tone language, we mean a language in which contrastive variations in pitch at the syllable level are used to distinguish the lexical or dictionary meaning of a word. Japanese and the other so-called *pitch-accent* languages of Europe are excluded by this definition. While this particular typological division is somewhat arbitrary, it is of little immediate consequence because of the lack of any published data, excepting Monrad-Krohn (1947), on the production of pitch-accent by aphasic speakers of such languages.

The aim of this chapter is to evaluate previously published findings that bear crucially on the production of tone in aphasia. Three major questions to be addressed are (1) To what extent is there a tone production deficit in aphasia? (2) What is the nature of the speech or language mechanisms

45

that underlie the tone production deficit? and (3) To what extent is the production of tone associated with left or right hemisphere specialization?

EXTENT OF TONE PRODUCTION DEFICIT IN APHASIA

At the time of this writing only 10 studies that provide any information on tone production in aphasia are available in the literature. All of these deal with aphasics who are native speakers of tone languages in the Far East: Mandarin Chinese, Cantonese, and Thai. No studies are available on aphasics who are native speakers of tone languages in other parts of the world, especially Africa and Central America. Nine are single case studies; one employs a group research methodology.

Four of the single case studies deal with bilingual aphasics. Lyman et al. (1938) reported that "spontaneous speech was natural" (p. 492) in both Mandarin Chinese and English for a patient with a lesion in the left occipitoparietal region. Thus, it may be inferred that their patient had no difficulty in producing the 4 lexical tones of Mandarin Chinese or any of their positional variants in connected speech. T'sou (1978) reported on a Cantonese–English bilingual conduction aphasic with a lesion in the left temporoparietal region. His patient had difficulty in producing only 1 of the 6 Cantonese tones, the *low falling* tone. The patient substituted the *low level* tone for the *low falling* tone in 5 of 7 productions of monosyllabic words in isolation. Two other studies involving bilingual Cantonese–English aphasics are cases of crossed aphasia. In their study of a right-handed male patient with a lesion in the right frontal region, April and Tse (1977) reported that his repetition of single Cantonese words was spared, but sentence repetition was severely impaired. Presumably, the 6 lexical tones of Cantonese were produced correctly in single word repetition. However, April and Tse were not able to provide any more information on tone production because of the paucity of their patient's Cantonese speech. In another study of a right-handed male patient with a lesion in the right frontal region, April and Han (1980) were similarly unable to provide any detailed information on tone production.

The remaining 5, single-case studies deal with monolingual aphasics. Two of the studies are with Chinese aphasics, 3 with Thai aphasics. Alajouanine and colleagues (1973) reported on a right-handed male Chinese Broca's aphasic with a lesion in the left hemisphere. Errors in tonal production occurred in his spontaneous speech. However, in repetition, his production of Mandarin tones was correct. In their study of a right-handed female Chinese global aphasic, Naeser and Chan (1980) reported that her production of Mandarin tones, especially the *low falling-rising* tone, was impaired in word repetition. On one of the repetition tests, she repeated the *low falling-rising* tone correctly on only 2 out of 15 trials. Interestingly, her production of Mandarin tones was less impaired in monosyllabic than in bisyllabic word repetition. Errors in tonal production also occurred in her spontaneous speech, elicited speech, object and picture naming, and Chinese character reading. Of the three published case studies of Thai aphasics, tone errors were reported to occur rarely in spontaneous speech, repetition, as well as other production-related tasks for a nonfamilial, left-handed, male conduction aphasic with major infraction in the left temporoparietal region (Gandour et al., 1982a), a right-handed male transcortical motor aphasic with a lesion in the left frontal region (Gandour et al., 1982b), and a right-handed female Broca's aphasic with a lesion in the left frontoparietal region (Gandour et al., 1985).

In his experimental study using a word repetition test, Packard (1986) found that right-handed Mandarin Chinese nonfluent aphasics with unilateral left hemisphere lesions (n = 8) experienced a deficit in tone production. As a group, Packard found that these aphasics' tone errors were similar both quantitatively and qualitatively to consonant errors. The mean error rate for tones was comparable to that for consonants; substitution errors predominated for both tones and consonants. As measured on phonological features, most tone and consonant errors reflected single feature substitutions.

There is a lack of convergence from these previously published data concerning the extent of the tone production deficit in aphasia. Because of these conflicting findings, it is important for us to re-evaluate some of the earlier studies in light of potentially confounding variables that may have had an effect on tone production. Two such variables that are of relevance here are the linguistic background of the patient and the time interval after his or her stroke.

Naeser and Chan (1980) described their patient as monolingual (Chinese) but tridialectal (Jiangxi province dialect, Mandarin, and Cantonese). From a linguistic perspective, their use of the term *dialect* is highly unorthodox. According to Naeser and Chan, their patient was not bilingual for Chinese and English, and therefore, was monolingual for the Chinese language. However, it is well-known that the various languages spoken in China such as Mandarin and Cantonese are referred to as dialects of Chinese because they are spoken within a single country and have a common writing system. In spoken form, Mandarin and Cantonese are mutually unintelligible languages. Indeed, Naeser and Chan themselves pointed out that "each dialect has its own phonological and tonal system" (p. 393). Therefore, their patient was apparently at least bilingual for Mandarin and Cantonese. No documentation was available for her native dialect spoken in Jiangxi province. Prior to her stroke, her husband, a native speaker of Cantonese, spoke to her mainly in Mandarin. Her children communicated with her in Cantonese. Naeser and Chan tested her in Mandarin, although it was not known how much she used Mandarin before her stroke. It is difficult to interpret her errors in tonal production because of this patient's complicated linguistic background, differences between the Mandarin and Cantonese tonal systems, lack of information about the tonal system of the Jiangxi province dialect, as well as uncertainty about the language she mainly used prior to her stroke. It is possible that her errors in producing Mandarin tones could be attributed to language or dialect interference instead of aphasia. Therefore, it is highly questionable that the Naeser and Chan study provides incontrovertible evidence that tone production is impaired in aphasics who are monolingual, native speakers of a tone language.

Based on findings for a group of nonfluent Mandarin Chinese aphasics, Packard (1986) has suggested that aphasic speakers of a tone language experience difficulty in producing tones that are both quantitatively and qualitatively equivalent to their difficulty in producing consonants. However, his group was quite heterogeneous in terms of months post-onset. Four of his subjects were tested within two months post-onset, four were tested more than 2 months post-onset. If error rates are computed for individual subjects, it is found that tone production errors were not distributed evenly among the eight aphasics. Of the total number of tone production errors, 74% were made by those 4 subjects who were tested within 2 months post-onset. Moreover, a Spearman rank order correlation analysis revealed that there was a significant negative relationship between the number of tone errors made by individual subjects and his or her time interval post-onset ($r_{ranks} = -.78$, $N = 8$, $p < .022$).

Time elapsed from onset is a very important factor in the study of aphasia. In general, patients are not neurologically or behaviorally stable until 2 to 3 months post-onset (Kertesz, 1979). Four of Packard's 8 subjects were tested within two months after the stroke. In our reanalysis of Packard's data, we have demonstrated that the extent of tonal disturbance may be related to the patient's stage of recovery. Tone production is less likely to be impaired in later stages of recovery. It is also possible that the tone production deficit of Packard's 4 subjects who were tested within 2 months after the stroke might be due to dysarthria instead of aphasia. Subjects with *minimal dysarthria* were not excluded from his group of nonfluent aphasics. At any rate, we can now reconcile the apparent conflict in findings between Packard's study and case studies by Gandour et al. (1982a, 1982b, 1985) of Thai aphasics. All three Thai aphasics were tested in later stages of recovery. The conduction aphasic was 9 years poststroke (Gandour et al., 1982a), the transcortical motor aphasic 4-1/2 years poststroke (Gandour et al., 1982b), and the Broca's aphasic 3 years poststroke (Gandour et al., 1985). None of these Thai patients exhibited any difficulty in producing the 5 Thai tones. Of special interest is the Broca's aphasic: "While the patient characteristically exhibited effortful and distorted articulation at the segmental level involving consonants and vowels, her ability to produce the 5 Thai tones remained intact" (Gandour et al., 1985, p. 553). Thus, it appears that a tone production deficit is manifested primarily in acute aphasic populations.

Because of the wide range of intersubject variability in Packard's group of left anterior aphasics, it may be unwise to represent their behavior by reporting only a group mean. As Caramazza and Martin (1983) have argued,

> Unlike the case of research with normal subjects, when evaluating group performance of aphasic patients, one cannot consider the within group variance as consisting primarily of random error variance but must seriously consider the possibility that a large part of this variance is caused by theoretically important individual difference. Consequently, special precautions should be taken when designing and interpreting aphasic research based upon group methodology (p. 27).

In the absence of such precautions in Packard's methodology, it is difficult to draw any firm conclusions concerning not only the extent of the tone production deficit, but also the extent to which it is quantitatively or qualitatively comparable to a consonant production deficit. Contrary to Packard's findings, Gandour and colleagues (1985) reported that the verbal output of their Thai Broca's aphasic indicates that tones and consonants may be disrupted independently. Consonant errors in syllable-initial position were frequent; vowel errors were not uncommon. Tone errors, on the other hand, were rare. In producing the 5 Thai tones, she totally ignored the phonological constraint of standard Thai which disallows *high* and *rising* tones on smooth syllables beginning with voiceless unaspirated stops. Thus, she produced the 5 tones without any regard for the segmental quality of the syllable-initial consonant. Despite deterioration of articulatory control of consonants and vowels, this patient maintained her phonatory control of the 5 Thai tones.

To the extent that there is a tone production deficit, the question arises about the extent to which the deficit is general or specific. Are tones impaired across the board? Or instead, are some tones spared while others are impaired? On a tone repetition test, Naeser and Chan's (1980) patient scored 88% correct for three (tones 1, 2, and 4) of the 4 Mandarin Chinese tones, but only 13% correct for the *low falling-rising* tone (tone 3). In fact, 72% of the total number of errors involved the *low falling-rising* tone. According to Naeser and Chan (1980), "she inconsistently substituted an unfamiliar, unidentifiable rising tone different from tone 2 and tone 3 words which could have been part of her original dialect, but which could not be confirmed" (p. 405). Interestingly, 52% of the total number of confusion errors in Packard's (1986) study were made in response to the Mandarin third tone (Packard, 1985, p. 86). Of these tone-3 confusion errors,

92% were substitutions of tone 2, the *mid-high rising* tone (Packard, 1985, p. 86). It may not be accidental that tone 3 appears to be less resistant to disruption in aphasia than the other 3 Mandarin Chinese tones. In comparison to tones 1, 2, and 4, tone 3 alone exhibits a complex bidirectional F_O contour. The fact that the tone that has the most complex F_O contour is the one most affected in aphasia suggests that the aphasic disturbance is of a phonetic nature. However, it is also possible that the aphasic disturbance is phonological in nature. Tone 3 and tone 2 are related by phonological rule. The Mandarin Chinese third tone always changes to tone 2, the *mid-high rising* tone, when immediately followed by another third tone. Problems of methodology notwithstanding, these findings from both the Naeser and Chan (1980) and Packard (1985, 1986) studies suggest that tones may be differentially susceptible to aphasic disturbance.

Moreover, it is possible that the lack of agreement in findings between the Mandarin Chinese and Thai aphasics may be related to differences in the tonal systems of Mandarin Chinese and Thai. Mandarin Chinese has four lexical tones; Thai has 5. The 5 Mandarin Chinese tones may be described phonetically as *high level* (tone 1), *mid-high rising* (tone 2), *low falling-rising* (tone 3), and *high falling* (tone 4); the five Thai tones as *mid level, low falling, high falling, high rising*, and *low rising*. Mandarin Chinese has several phonological rules that bring about tonal substitutions in connected speech; Thai does not. Tones could be differentially resistant to impairment depending on the number of tones in the phonemic inventory, the distribution of their F_O trajectories in the tone space, and the kinds of phonological processes they undergo.

NATURE OF TONE PRODUCTION DEFICIT IN APHASIA

Due to the paucity of data on tone production in aphasia, only two hypotheses that are relevant to this issue are explicit enough to warrant discussion. By one hypothesis, the tone production deficit is conceptualized as a lexical–phonological disorder. By the other hypothesis, the tone production deficit is conceptualized primarily as a timing problem in larger-sized linguistic units. Deterioration of tones is secondary to dissolution of temporal structure. Although we are not able to resolve this issue conclusively at the time of this writing, it is important that we evaluate these two hypotheses. In so doing, we will conclude that only the second hypothesis is likely to serve as a useful guide for future research.

Based on his findings for a group of left anterior Mandarin Chinese aphasics, Packard (1986) hypothesized that the tone production deficit lies in the lexicon. According to Packard, it is a lexical disorder because only idiosyncratic, nonredundant information is specified in the lexicon. The phonological information that must be listed in the lexicon is just that which is not predictable from context. Thus, phonemic information about consonants, vowels, and tones is provided in the lexicon. Assuming that the lexicon is under the control of the left hemisphere, Packard argues that the tonal deficit in left anterior aphasics follows from the fact that tonal information is specified in the lexicon.

Packard's hypothesis implies that a disruption at the phonetic surface that involves phonologically contrastive units should coincide with a disruption of phonological information in the lexicon. If the phonetic manifestation of lexical consonants, vowels, or tones is aberrant, it is predicted that the phonological contrast will not be preserved. Ignoring the distinction between phonetic and phonological levels of processing, Packard's hypothesis cannot handle those cases in which phonology is preserved in spite of deviant phonetics. Such cases are not uncommon in the aphasia literature. For example, in their study of Thai aphasics' productions of phonologically contrastive short and long vowels, Gandour and Dardarananda (1984) found that the relative temporal relationship between short and long vowels was preserved despite deviant, absolute duration values.

By focusing on the lexicon as the source of the tonal deficit, it is not at all clear how Packard can account for the dichotomy between phonetic and phonemic patterns of dissolution in Broca's and Wenicke's aphasia. Moreover, the production deficit in Broca's aphasia is generally assumed to reflect difficulty both at the level of articulatory implementation and phonemic selection. In this sense, it is both phonetic and phonological in nature (cf. Blumstein et al., 1980). Yet, Packard treats the tonal deficit in Broca's aphasia as if it were purely phonological in nature. Further, any dissociation between consonants, vowels, and tones in terms of a production deficit, either quantitatively or qualitatively, is left unaccounted for at the lexical level of processing (cf. Gandour et al., 1985).

With attention to acoustic phonetics and syntax, Danly and Shapiro's (1982) investigation of dysprosody in Broca's aphasia provides a much more promising point of departure for research into the nature of the tone production deficit in aphasia. In their study of five English-speaking Broca's aphasics, Danly and Shapiro demonstrated that a simple characterization of dysprosody in Broca's aphasia was in need of revision. Using three acoustic measures of speech prosody—sentence-final F_O fall, declination of F_O peaks throughout a sentence, sentence-final segmental lengthening—they found that some aspects of prosody were spared while others were abnormal. All Broca's aphasics, regardless of degree of impairment, exhibited sentence final F_O fall. F_O declination was present in short sentences, but absent in longer sentences. Sentence-final lengthening was absent; in fact, sentence-final words were actually shorter than their sentence-initial and sentence-medial counterparts. Broca's aphasics, in addition, reset F_O contours in longer sentences more often than normal subjects. These findings led Danly and Shapiro to hypothesize that Broca's aphasics have a narrower-than-normal scope for linguistic planning.

F_O declination appears only within shorter sentences because syntactic planning units are shorter in Broca's aphasics. Because intonation production necessarily involves sentence- or phrase-sized units, it remains to be determined if it is only when higher level syntactic planning is involved that a deficit in F_O production occurs. To help clarify this issue, F_O production needs to be investigated in word-sized units, where phonetic processing has not interacted with syntactic processing. F_O production deficits at the word or syllable level would point to a lower level phonological or phonetic disorder. Ryalls (1984) analyzed properties of F_O in single-word utterances produced by English-speaking aphasics. The F_O of anterior aphasics was significantly higher than that of normal speakers; the difference in F_O between the posterior aphasics and the normal speakers was not. Both groups of aphasics showed increased variability in F_O as compared to normal speakers. Such findings suggest that we need to distinguish between phonetic and phonological factors in F_O disintegration following damage to the brain. Extending this line of research, what needs to be investigated is F_O production that corresponds to a feature of linguistic structure at the word level. Such a prosodic feature is tone.

Take, for example, Thai, a tone language with 5 contrastive tones. F_O variations are phonologically contrastive at the level of the syllable. If we assume that (1) the syllable is the minimal unit of timing in speech production; (2) Broca's aphasics have a limited capacity to plan speech over larger-sized linguistic units; and (3) the scope for linguistic planning in Thai-speaking Broca's aphasics is intact within the boundaries of a syllable, then we should expect Thai-speaking Broca's aphasics to be able to produce tonal contrasts successfully in monosyllabic citation forms. If control of F_O and timing are independent, then we should further expect F_O patterns to be preserved within syllables when they occur in polysyllabic words, phrases, and sentences in spite of abnormal timing patterns between syllables. If so, such data would provide support for the notion that dysprosody in Broca's aphasia is not solely a manifestation of articulatory or phonatory difficulties, but instead a manifestation of timing difficulties over larger-sized linguistic units. Such acoustic phonetic studies have yet to be completed in Thai or any other tone language.

With this different conceptualization of dysprosody in Broca's aphasia, it may be inappropriate to speak of a tone production deficit per se. It is not the control of F_O that is in question, but rather the control of F_O over a specified time interval. The critical variable is the size of the domain over which the prosodic patterns extend. By definition, intonational patterns extend over larger-sized linguistic units when compared to tonal patterns. If dysprosody in Broca's aphasia is primarily due to a narrower-than-normal scope for linguistic planning, it is predicted that tones will be more resistant to disruption than intonation. To produce intonation successfully, one must be able to control timing over sentence-

or phrase-sized units; to produce tones successfully, one must be able to control timing over word- or syllable-sized units. Deviant timing at the sentence level necessarily disrupts F_O contours associated with intonations. Whereas, in a tone language, deviant timing at the sentence level does not necessarily disrupt F_O contours associated with tones. By undertaking investigations of the production of tone, intonation, and other aspects of prosody in aphasia, we will bring ourselves a step closer to understanding the nature of the tone production deficit. In so doing, the Danly–Shapiro hypothesis provides a single mechanism that can account for similarities and differences in speech prosody in aphasia across languages.

It must also be noted that the phonetic shapes of tones may vary as a function of the immediate tonal context, sentence position, stress, and intonation (Ho, 1976; 1977; Abramson, 1979a; 1979b; Abramson & Svastikula, 1983). Although the contrasts between the tones is preserved, their shapes are not identical to those that appear in citation forms of monosyllabic words. Whether or not such perturbations of the F_O contours through tonal coarticulation, sentence position, stress, and intonation are maintained in aphasic speech is an important topic for future research. If the shapes of the F_O contours deteriorate in these larger-sized linguistic units, we will have strong evidence that dysprosody in aphasia is primarily due to faulty control of timing instead of F_O.

HEMISPHERIC SPECIALIZATION FOR TONE PRODUCTION

As with other linguistic units and levels of processing, evidence concerning the lateralization of lexical tone may provide insights into the representation of language in the human brain. Are tones lateralized to the left hemisphere, to the right hemisphere, or are they instead, bilaterally represented? With regard to tone perception, dichotic listening studies on the perception of Thai tones by normal speakers (Van Lancker & Fromkin, 1973; 1978) and tone identification tests with left and right brain-damaged Thai patients (Gandour & Dardarananda, 1983) and Mandarin Chinese patients (Naeser and Chan, 1980; Hughes et al., 1983; Packard, 1985) indicate that the perception of tone is lateralized to the left hemisphere. With regard to tone production, data are scarce and often difficult to interpret because of methodological problems. Moreover, detailed acoustic phonetic studies have yet to be completed with aphasics who are speakers of a tone language. We can nevertheless bring the issues into sharper focus by evaluating the evidence presently available, and thereby establish directions for future research.

A tone-production deficit secondary to a lesion in the right hemisphere has not yet been reported in the literature for monolingual speakers of tone languages. In those studies reporting a tone production deficit, all patients have had unilateral left-hemisphere lesions. (Naeser & Chan, 1980; Packard, in press). Conversely, Hughes et al. (1983) reported that none of their 12 patients with unilateral right-hemisphere lesions had any difficulty in producing the four Mandarin Chinese tones. Although patients who had lesions on the opposite side were not included in either the Packard (1986) or Hughes et al. (1983) investigation, their findings together indicate that the tone production deficit may be restricted to left brain-damaged patients. At the same time, we cannot dismiss entirely the possibility of a right-hemisphere contribution to the production of tone. Right-hemisphere damage has recently been shown to affect the production of lexical stress, contrastive stress, and intonation patterns in English (Weintraub et al., 1981; Shapiro & Danly, 1985). Such findings suggest that right hemisphere damage may affect prosodic features of speech in a more general manner than was previously assumed. Consequently, we cannot maintain the position that the production of tones is lateralized to the left hemisphere simply because tones are part of the linguistic system.

As an alternative hypothesis, Van Lancker (1980) has recently proposed a scale of hemispheric specialization associated with different domains (segment, syllable, word, phrase, and sentence) of functional pitch contrasts. The scale ranges from *most linguistically structured* pitch contrasts (e.g., Thai tone, and Japanese word accent) associated with left hemispheric specialization to *least linguistically structured* pitch contrasts (e.g., emotional tone, and personal voice quality) associated with right hemisphere specialization. That is, hemispheric specialization is determined by the extent to which F_O patterns are linguistic. One obvious problem with Van Lancker's formulation is how to decide in a principled, nonarbitrary manner precisely where to draw the boundary lines along this linguistic continuum. Another problem is that although the domains associated with different F_O patterns are mentioned, Van Lancker focuses primarily on linguistic function. Temporal differences between the different domains are ignored. Without taking the temporal characteristics of the domains into account, Van Lancker's proposal cannot accommodate those aphasic patients whose ability to produce a given prosodic pattern varies depending upon the length of utterance.

According to Packard (1985), "it is not solely *whether* an entity participates in the linguistic system, or even the *extent* to which it participates, but that it is rather the *nature* of its participation in the linguistic system that determines the hemispheric lateralization of that entity" (p. 105). The issue then becomes what differences in nature of participation in the linguistic system are correlated with differences in hemispheric specialization. As discussed in earlier sections of this chapter, Packard's lexical–postlexical distinction fails to make the right predictions in several different cases of aphasic disturbance of speech prosody.

There is an intimate relationship between the control of F_O and timing. Using acoustic phonetic measures of intonation and rhythm in aphasic speech, Danly and her colleagues (1982; 1983) have clearly demonstrated that the programming of F_O crucially depends on sentence length, and further, that the programming of F_O may be less disrupted than the programming of timing. These findings are compatible with the notion that the left hemisphere is specialized for temporal analysis. The programming of F_O necessarily intersects with temporal planning in sentence production. Thus, disruption of F_O contours does not necessarily indicate a malfunction in F_O mechanisms, but instead a secondary effect due to a malfunction in timing mechanisms. Based on the data currently available in the literature, we can only speculate that tones will be less disrupted than intonation because of the smaller temporal domain over which they extend. It is important to keep in mind, however, that even though tonal contrasts may be preserved, there might still be phonetic deterioration due to the absence of coarticulatory influences on the shape of F_O contours that are present in normal speech. The presence versus absence of tonal coarticulation may indeed turn out to be diagnostically significant in distinguishing between anterior and posterior aphasic syndromes. By analyzing the tone production deficit within a temporal context, it is expected that we will significantly increase our understanding of the production of tone, as well as other aspects of prosody, in aphasia.

CONCLUSIONS

Unfortunately, this review of earlier published studies concerning a tone production deficit in aphasia does not allow us to come to a definite resolution of the three major questions addressed in this chapter. Because of limited data, conflicting findings, methodological problems in a few frequently cited studies, and most importantly, the absence of any acoustic phonetic investigations, we have seen that even the extent of the tone production deficit in aphasia remains an open question. Not until such investigations are undertaken can we ever hope to resolve these questions concerning tone production in aphasia. Indeed, it wasn't until very recently that acoustic phonetic studies have begun to illuminate the phonological and phonetic characteristics of aphasics' productions of consonants (e.g., Blumstein et al., 1980), vowels (e.g., Ryalls, 1986), and intonation (e.g., Danly & Shapiro, 1982). Tone languages offer some research opportunities that cannot be duplicated in nontone languages. The fact that lexical tones are defined over the domain of a single syllable provides us with an especially clear window for looking into the possible dissociation of control of F_O and timing. At the time of this writing, we can only look forward to the completion of such studies.

REFERENCES

Abramson, A.S. (1979a). Lexical tone and sentence prosody in Thai. In E. Fischer-Jorgensen, J. Rischel, & N. Thorsen (Eds.), *Proceedings of the Ninth International Congress of Phonetic Sciences* (Vol. II), Copenhagen: University of Copenhagen, (pp. 380–387).

Abramson, A.S. (1979b). The coarticulation of tones: An acoustic study of Thai. In V. Panupong, P. Kullavanijaya, K. Tingsabadh, & T. Luangthongkum (Eds.), *Studies of Tai and Mon-Khmer phonetics in honour of Eugenie J.A. Henderson.* Bangkok: Chulalongkorn University Press, pp. 1–9.

Abramson, A.S., & Svastikula, K. (1983). Intersections of tone and intonation in `Thai (Status Report on Speech Research SR-74/75), New Haven, CT: Haskins Laboratories, pp. 143–154.

Alajouanine, R., Cathala, H.P., Metellus, J., Siksou, M., Alleton, V., Cheng, F., DeTurckheim, C., & Chang, M.C. (1973). La problématique de l'aphasie dans les langues à écriture non-alphabetique: A propos d'un cas chez un Chinois. *Revue Neurologique, 128,* 229–243.

April, R.S., & Han, M. (1980). Crossed aphasia in a right-handed bilingual Chinese man, a second case. *Archives of Neurology, 37,* 342–346.

April, R.S., & Tse, P.C. (1977). Crossed aphasia in a Chinese bilingual dextral. *Archives of Neurology, 34,* 766–770.

Blumstein, S., Cooper, W., Goodglass, H., Statlender, S., & Gottlieb, J. (1980). Production deficits in aphasia: A voice-onset-time analysis. *Brain and Language, 9,* 153–170.

Caramazza, A., & Martin, R.C. (1983). Theoretical and methodological issues in the study of aphasia. In J.B. Hellige (Ed.), *Cerebral hemisphere asymmetry: Method, theory, and application* New York: Praeger, pp. 18–45.

Cooper, W.E., Soares, C., Nicol, J., Michelou, D. & Goloskie, S. (1984). Clausal intonation after unilateral brain damage. *Language and Speech, 27,* 17–24.

Cooper, W.E., and Sorensen, J.M. (1981). *Fundamental frequency in sentence production.* New York: Springer-Verlag.

Danly, M., Cooper, W.E., & Shapiro, B. (1983). Fundamental frequency, language processing, and linguistic structure in Wernicke's aphasia. *Brain and Language, 19,* 1–24.

Danly, M., & Shapiro, B. (1982). Speech prosody in Broca's aphasia. *Brain and Language, 16,* 171–190.

Gandour, J., Buckingham, H., Jr., Dardarananda, R., Stawathumrong, P., & Petty, S. (1982a). Case study of a Thai conduction aphasic. *Brain and Language, 17,* 327–358.

Gandour, J., & Dardarananda, R. (1983). Identification of tonal contrasts in Thai aphasic patients. *Brain and Language, 18,* 98–114.

Gandour, J., & Dardarananda, R. (1984). Prosodic disturbance in aphasia: Vowel length in Thai. *Brain and Language, 23,* 206–224.

Gandour, J., Dardarananda, R., & Vejjajiva, A. (1985). Case study of a Thai Broca aphasic with an adaptation of the Boston Diagnostic Aphasia Examination. *Journal of the Medical Association of Thailand, 68,* 552–563.

Gandour, J., Dardarananda, R., Vibulsreth, S., & Buckingham, H., Jr., (1982b).

Case study of a Thai transcortical motor aphasic. *Language and Speech, 25,* 127–150.

Ho, A.T. (1976). The acoustic variation of Mandarin tones. *Phonetica, 33,* 353–367.

Ho, A.T. (1977). Intonation variation in a Mandarin sentence for three expressions: Interrogative, exclamatory, and declarative. *Phonetica, 34,* 446–457.

Hughes, C.P., Chan, J.L., & Ming, S.S. (1983). Aprosodia in Chinese patients with right cerebral hemisphere lesion. *Archives of Neurology, 40,* 732–736.

Kent, R.D., & Rosenbek, J.C. (1983). Acoustic patterns of apraxia of speech. *Journal of Speech and Hearing Research, 26,* 231–249.

Kertesz, A. (1979). *Aphasia and associated disorders: Taxonomy, localization, and recovery.* New York: Grune & Stratton.

Lyman, R.S., Kwan, S.T., & Chao, W.H. (1938). Left occipito parietal brain tumor with observations on alexia and agraphia in Chinese and in English. *Chinese Medical Journal, 54,* 491–516.

Monrad-Krohn, G.H. (1947). Dysprosody or altered melody of language. *Brain, 70,* 405–423.

Naeser, M.A., & Chan, S.W.C. (1980). Case study of a Chinese aphasic with the Boston Diagnostic Aphasia Exam. *Neuropsychologia, 18,* 389–410.

Packard, J.L. (1985). A linguistic investigation of tone laterality in aphasic Chinese speakers. (Doctoral dissertation, Cornell University, 1984) *Dissertation Abstracts International, 45,* 2860A.

Packard, J.L. (1986). Tone production deficits in non-fluent aphasic Chinese speech. *Brain and Language, 29,* 212–223.

Ryalls, J.H. (1984). Some acoustic aspects of fundamental frequency of CVC utterances in aphasia. *Phonetica, 41,* 103–111.

Ryalls, J.H. (1986). A study of vowel production in aphasia. *Brain and Language, 29,* 48–67.

Shapiro, B.E., & Danly, M. (1985) The role of the right hemisphere in the control of speech prosody in propositional and affective contexts. *Brain and Language, 25,* 19–36.

T'sou, B.K. (1978). Some preliminary observations on aphasia in a Chinese bilingual. *Acta Psychologica Taiwanica, 20,* 57–64.

Van Lancker, D. (1980). Cerebral lateralization of pitch cues in the linguistic signal. *Papers in Linguistics, 13*(2), 201–277.

Van Lancker, D., & Fromkin, V.A. (1973). Hemispheric specialization for pitch and tone: Evidence from Thai. *Journal of Phonetics, 1,* 101–109.

Van Lancker, D., & Fromkin, V.A. (1978). Cerebral dominance for pitch contrasts in tone language speakers and in musically untrained and trained English speakers. *Journal of Phonetics, 6,* 19–23.

Weintraub, S., Mesulam, M., & Kramer, L. (1981). Disturbances in prosody: A right hemisphere contribution to language. *Archives of Neurology, 38,* 742–744.

C H A P T E R 4

Intonation in Aphasic and Right-Hemisphere-Damaged Patients

William E. Cooper
Gayle V. Klouda

Intonational aspects of speech have been utilized traditionally to help characterize and distinguish various aphasic disorders. Generally, intonation refers to speech variations in time, amplitude, and fundamental voice frequency (hereafter F_o, often referred to by its perceptual correlate, *voice pitch*) that are superimposed over the segments of speech. The communicative functions of intonation are manifold and include conveying emotional tone (e.g., Williams & Stevens, 1972; Cosmides, 1983), linguistic stress (e.g., as in distinguishing the noun and verb forms of *convict*), varying degrees of emphasis among different words in a sentence (e.g., Selkirk, 1984; Cooper, Eady, & Mueller, 1985), and syntactic structure (e.g., Lea, 1973; Cooper & Sorensen, 1981).

Interest in intonational aspects of aphasia stems historically from the observation by Broca (1861) that lesions in the third frontal convolution of the left hemisphere were accompanied by speech dysfluency. The speech of Broca's aphasics is typified by numerous interword pauses, sometimes as long as a few seconds. The clinical impression of dysfluency has customarily played a major role in characterizing Broca's aphasia in neuropsychological examinations (e.g. Goodglass & Kaplan, 1972; Wagenaar, Snow, & Prins, 1975; Demeurisse, et al., 1979; Kreindleer, Mihailescu, & Fradis, 1980). In this vein, Broca's dysfluent speech is contrasted with the generally fluent output of Wernicke's aphasics.

In the past 15 years, the study of intonation in aphasia has been illuminated by two technological advances, involving computerized acoustical analysis techniques and computerized neuroimaging. With the help of these techniques, impressionistic observations that have traditionally been quite useful in clinical settings can now be supplemented by measures that are more precise and reliable. At the same time, studies of speech perception have indicated that the human hearer does not perceive speech in a manner that is always in direct correspondence with the acoustical signal, underscoring the need for objective measures that go beyond the unaided ear (e.g., Lieberman, 1965; Martin, 1970; Breckenridge, 1977). For the most part, the following sections will focus on studies that have utilized such objective techniques to examine the intonational attributes of F_O and duration.

In addition to technological advances, the study of intonation in aphasia has been enhanced by modern theoretical developments in cognitive psychology. In particular, models of information-processing have emphasized issues of information routing, independence of subprocesses, sites of interaction, and similar topics that can be studied in aphasia with reference to how intonation is programmed by the speaker. For example, is intonation programmed independently of lexical selection, such that aphasic errors in lexical choice are independent of intonational errors? In a similar vein, theoretical work on aphasia typology has suggested that the distinctions between traditional subtypes like Broca's and Wernicke's aphasia might be superceded by more fundamental distinctions, including the distinction between automatic and controlled information-processing (e.g., Blumstein & Milberg, 1983). It is no longer the case that Broca's aphasia is considered to be exclusively a motor problem, nor Wernicke's aphasia exclusively a sensory one (e.g., Danly, Cooper, & Shapiro, 1983). But it is not yet possible to unravel the nature of which distinctions are most fundamental. The problem here is compounded by the fact that lesion sites themselves are seldom "pure," often involving more than a single functional area. Especially in the case of intonation, other complications involving emotional state can influence speech output, making the task of isolating linguistically relevant sites of damage difficult. But for purposes of exposition, the traditional dichotomy between Broca's and Wernicke's aphasia will be utilized here as a simple means of grouping various studies.

Many early studies precategorized aphasic subgroups by neurological and neuropsychological examination in terms of these traditional categories, then looked for differences in intonation. Now, the possibility of larger sample sizes and more standardized neuroimaging data allows for the investigator to conduct a "blind" study of intonation on all patients admitted on the basis of aphasia, allowing for more information to be obtained on new subtypes and special cases, including subcortical aphasics. Given the potential complications involved in aphasic samples, one would ideally want to include a much larger sample of aphasics in each group than is typical in experimentation with normal subjects. However, most aphasics studies of necessity utilize a much smaller sample, making interpretation especially risky in comparison with brain-behavior studies of animals that take advantage of the fact that many nonlanguage tasks can be successfully modeled in other species.

BROCA'S APHASIA

The speech of Broca's aphasics has been clinically described as sounding intonationally flat (e.g., Goodglass & Kaplan, 1972). This perception is substantiated in two recent studies reporting a somewhat restricted F_O range for Broca's when compared to the speech of normals (Ryalls, 1982; Cooper et al., 1984). In Ryalls' study, 8 Broca's aphasics, all native speakers of French, produced a single sentence "Construisons notre maison," and their productions were compared with those of 11 normal subjects. The subjects were asked to repeat this sentence after a clinician, and the tape recorded utterances of the clinician were then used for the normal subjects as well to negate any effects of mimicry. F_O estimates were obtained by extrapolating from the values of the fifth harmonic of narrow-band spectrograms. Ryalls measured the highest and lowest frequency of a steady state portion of F_O (he does not indicate criteria of "steady state"). The difference between these two measures was then taken as the F_O range.

In this particular study, the mean F_O was comparable for the two groups (cf. Ryalls, Chapter 2, for other work indicating higher mean F_O for Broca's aphasics in other studies), whereas the F_O range was significantly more restricted for the Broca's aphasics. In addition, the utterance durations were significantly longer for the Broca's aphasics. Ryalls suggested that this F_O compression might be accounted for by a depletion of pulmonary air pressure, needed for the prolonged production of Broca's speech. Aside from compression of the overall peak to valley F_O range, a study of English-speaking aphasics has revealed a compression in the differences among F_O peaks for Broca's aphasics in comparison with normals (Cooper et al., 1984).

In contrast, Danly and Shapiro (1982) reported exaggerated rather than restricted F_O modulation for Broca's aphasics. They measured F_O variation by summing valley-peak-valley F_O differences on selected key words embedded within sentences. While, as Ryalls (1986b) points out, their results appear to contradict both the clinical impressions of flat intonation for this patient group and the acoustic results reported by Ryalls (1982) and Cooper et al. (1984), there are several possible explanations for the apparent inconsistency. First, Danly and Shapiro's measure of F_O variation is a within-word, peak-to-valley index of variation, while Ryalls (1982) measured peak-to-valley fluctuation across sentences. Thus, the perception of flat intonation in Broca's speech may be based on restricted word-to-word F_O variation, while within-word variability may actually be increased. It is also possible that the apparent contradiction in results reflects a high degree of intersubject or intrasubject variability with respect to intonational fluctuations. As with many other key issues to be outlined here, clarification of this point will require further study with larger samples and careful analyses of information regarding lesion site.

Because the speech of Broca's aphasics is so manifestly nonfluent, one might question whether such patients retain any of the rudiments of normal speech prosody. This possibility was examined in two recent acoustical studies (Danly, deVilliers, & Cooper, 1979; Danly & Shapiro, 1982). Danly et al., 1979 examined the speech of Broca's utilizing two-word utterances, including those spoken spontaneously and those uttered in oral reading. In this and subsequently described oral reading tests, the patients were instructed to avoid the use of contrastive or emphatic stress while reading the sentences. When the patient grossly misarticulated a content word or exhibited unusual stress, he was asked to repeat the sentence until a satisfactory utterance was produced. In the case of Broca's speech, agrammatic speech output was acceptable as data, and, in the case of Wernicke's aphasics, paraphasias and neologisms were acceptable as long as the output utterance contained the same number of content words as the target utterance. With these provisions, one could analyze the difference between target and output for these aphasic groups in order to determine isolated and interactive aspects of their computational deficits.

Danly et al. (1979) analyzed the utterances for three prosodic characteristics that would ordinarily distinguish two-word from single-word utterances in normal speech. These features include a terminal falling contour of fundamental frequency on the second word from peak to valley, the declining of F_O peaks from the first word to the second, and an elongation of the second word. Of these attributes, the two-word utterances of Broca's aphasics reliably exhibited both a terminal falling F_O contour and F_O declination. On the other hand, the duration of the first of the two words was longer than that of the second word, contrary to findings for normal adults and children (Branigan, 1976a, 1976b; Danly & Shapiro, 1982). The same pattern of results was obtained in a comparison of the second and third words of three-word utterances spoken by Broca's aphasics in an oral reading test (Danly & Shapiro, 1982), suggesting that the lengthening of the first word in two-word utterances was not entirely attributable to a start-up effect in producing this word with heightened stress (cf. Goodglass, Fodor, & Schulhoff, 1967). It seems rather, that the difference in duration between the last word of the utterance and the next-to-last word is attributable to an abnormal shortening of the utterance-final word, accompanied by unusually low amplitude in many cases. Following Ryalls (1982), depletion of pulmonary air pressure might account for this effect. In longer utterances, however, it appears that Broca's aphasics utterance-final words are comparable in duration to normals, suggesting that Broca's aphasics regain pulmonary air via breathing before the ends of relatively long utterances (Cooper et al., 1984).

The fact that Broca's aphasics produce a larger terminal F_O fall on the last word of an utterance, despite producing a short-word duration is consistent with the view that utterance-final lengthening in normal speech is probably not produced in order to allow time for a large terminal F_O fall (cf., Klatt, 1975; Lyberg, 1979). The dissociation between utterance-final duration and F_O effects for the Broca's aphasics is consistent with the finding that, in normal speech, there exists no strong correlation in individual utterances between the amount of utterance-final lengthening and the amount of terminal F_O fall at major syntactic boundaries (Cooper & Sorensen, 1977; 1981). It appears that, while the programming of timing and F_O information is considered jointly at some high-level stage of processing, the programming of specific durations and F_O values proceed largely independent of one another.

Aside from the findings for duration, the F_O results reported by Danly et al. (1979) reveal that Broca's aphasics do retain some of the basic attributes of normal speech prosody, even though these characteristics are typically camouflaged by their very slow rate of speech and numerous large interword pauses. To the clinical ear, the speech of Broca's aphasics would no doubt seem much improved, albeit still abnormal, if it was tape recorded and then represented after someone had excised some of the more lengthy pauses. In this study, relatively normal terminal F_O fall and declination were observed despite interword pauses that averaged more than 1 second and included pauses as long as 7 seconds. No significant correlation was obtained between the length of these interword pauses and the magnitude or presence of the normal F_O attributes.

To further examine the F_O characteristics of Broca's aphasics, Danly & Shapiro (1982) conducted oral reading tests using longer sentence strings, ranging from 7 to 14 words each. The sentences had originally been tested with normals to investigate the mathematical form of F_O declination as well as the slope of declination in short versus long utterances (Cooper & Sorensen, 1981). An example sentence pair bearing on this latter issue is presented below. The italicized words represent stressed words, common to both sentences, measured for peak F_O.

The *cat* was *asleep* in the *tree*.
The *cat* that Sally owned was asleep on the large branch in the *tree*.

In their study of normal speech, Cooper and Sorensen found that speakers produced higher F_O peaks on the first stressed word of an utterance in long versus short sentences, presumably in order to allow a greater range for F_O declination in long utterances. In the study of Broca's speech using the same sentence materials, however, Danly and Shapiro (1982) found that the aphasics failed to produce higher F_O peaks in longer strings, unlike a group of nonneurological hospitalized control patients. These results suggest that Broca's aphasics do not consider the general length of a sentence when programming F_O in oral reading. This inference is consistent with their very limited capability to produce multiple word sentences. In addition, such patients did not show the same gradual trend of declining F_O peaks throughout the course of such utterances. Rather, the Broca's aphasics seemed to produce declination over 2 or 3 word phrases, and to reset their declination function many times within the sentence (especially for longer sentences), suggesting that their programming of F_O is carried out over domains that are much shorter than normal. The resetting generally respected syntactic boundaries, however, rarely occurring within the confines of phrasal units. Thus, Broca's aphasics seem to retain some degree of syntactic integrity in their speech, although it is also possible that this feature can be linked to intact semantic processing, a question for future study.

Danly and Shapiro (1982) further noted that the patients partially compensated for their halting speech by typically ending words within each phrase with a sizable continuation rise in F_O. The continuation rises produced by such patients do appear to warrant the description "compensatory", inasmuch as their frequency of occurrence and magnitude are greater than normal yet are quite appropriate given the shorter-than-normal domains of production with lengthy interword pauses. The frequency of continuation rises was positively correlated with the severity of language disorder across the 5 patients tested. Whether or not the Broca's speaker intends to aid the listener by producing these continuation rises, such rises undoubtedly serve this function, possibly in addition to helping the speaker demarcate his own units of processing. The effective utilization of continuation rises at the ends of words in Broca's speech seems to represent one aspect of a general tendency for these patients to exhibit more sophisticated control over F_O during the middle and final portions of a word than at or near a word's beginning. A closer examination of the F_O contours is needed at various locations within words to investigate this possibility further, but, if substantiated, Broca's difficulty in controlling F_O at the *beginnings* of words may be attributed to their need to devote so much of their processing at this point to motor commands associated with producing a correct phonemic representation of the first phoneme of a word, a region of special difficulty in the speech of such patients

(Goodglass et al., 1967). This possibility rests on the assumption that, although the detailed programming of F_O and phonemic representations are largely independent, a general executive of limited processing capacity may simplify or abandon certain F_O programming operations when the demands on processing phonemic representations are at a premium.

The presence of large and frequent continuation rises also provides the first piece of convincing evidence in favour of the notion that Broca's speakers plan for an upcoming word before completely executing a current one. Originally, the presence of declination and terminal F_O fall were taken as evidence in favor of this view (Danly et al., 1979; Danly & Shapiro, 1982), but a closer examination of these phenomena reveal problems with this interpretation. According to the notion that these patients program F_O over a span of at least 2 words, the speaker preplans an F_O contour for the 2 words prior to the uttering of either, complete with declining F_O peaks and terminal F_O fall. But, according to another alternative, the patient might not be endowed with such preplanning capability, but rather produces a default F_O contour for the first word, and only after uttering this word might the patient program F_O for a subsequent word. According to this alternative, the speaker must simply recognize when he or she is about to utter the terminal word of an utterance, programming a low-peak F_O and terminal falling pattern for this word. Such recognition could be delayed until just before the terminal word is spoken.

On the basis of declination and terminal F_O alone, it is difficult to distinguish between these two possible accounts. Both models predict, for example, that an analysis of single-word utterances would show F_O patterns similar to those of utterance-final words. Ideally, we would like to know exactly what the speaker preplans before the utterance has already been initiated and what the speaker plans thereafter, and an answer to this question must await research in which acoustical measures are combined with a task sensitive to the distinction between preplanning and planning-cum-execution, such as reaction time to initiate speech (see Cooper & Ehrlich, 1981).

The continuation rises that appear at the ends of nonterminal words, do suggest however, that Broca's speakers *are* capable of planning for an upcoming word. While it remains a possibility that such planning does not take place until some portion of a current word has been produced, continuation rises would not be expected if these speakers did not begin to plan for an upcoming word until the current word was completely uttered. In effect, then, the presence of strong continuation rises at the ends of nonterminal words in Broca's speech can be taken as evidence that some planning capabilities do span a unit encompassing more than a single word. What remains to be determined is whether such planning can take place for the patients even before the first word of an utterance is spoken.

To summarize, the Danly et al. studies (1979, 1982) of Broca's speech indicate that a few rudimentary attributes of normal F_O patterns are preserved in short utterances despite lengthy interword pauses and laboured articulation. On the other hand, these aphasics do not exhibit utterance-final lengthening as in normal speech, and Broca's speech is marked by evidence of shorter-than-normal domains of prosodic programming. The results imply a deficit in speech planning, but the extent to which this deficit is incurred before the initiation of speech or after initiation remains unknown. Additionally, it remains to be determined whether the planning domain available to Broca's aphasics is more properly characterized in terms of syntactic or semantic and pragmatic representations, but these questions can be addressed in future work using the same testing procedures.

As for the traditional clinical view that Broca's aphasics exhibit dysprosody, it now appears that this description is more applicable to speech timing—including both the durations of segments and pauses—than to fundamental frequency. While segmental timing in even short two-word utterances shows abnormally short durations of the utterance-final word and long interword pauses, fundamental frequency analysis shows at least a few normal characteristics, including the declining of F_O peaks from the first word to the second, and a terminal F_O fall from peak to valley in the utterance-final word. In addition, Broca's patients exhibit an ability to compensate in part for their shorter-than-normal domains of F_O declination by producing substantial continuation rises in F_O at the ends of utterance nonfinal words, signifying the intent to continue speaking. This highly adaptive employment of F_O suggests that these patients retain a rather sophisticated ability to program this prosodic attribute on the basis of higher-order considerations. Yet, because such control of F_O is not readily discerned by the clinical ear, when camouflaged by the very slow, halting rate of speech, so the impression of dysprosody is understandable. It is equally apparent, however, that the continued use of the term *dysprosody* is somewhat misleading insofar as it commonly connotes a primary deficit in the programming of F_O.

Although speech timing appears relatively more disturbed than F_O in Broca's speech, recent results suggest that some aspects of normal timing may also be preserved for some patients. Ryalls (1982) reported that Broca's exhibit both longer sentence durations and longer segment (vowel) durations when compared to normal speakers, but he failed to find significant group differences for mean vowel duration in a recent study of speech production including 5 anterior aphasics, 7 posterior aphasics, and 7 normal control subjects (Ryalls, 1986a). The Broca's did exhibit significantly greater variability in vowel duration, however. In another recent study, Williams and Seaver (1986) compared vowel and consonant durations produced by 3 groups of aphasics and a normal control group. They again found no significant differences for segment durations across groups. However, two

Broca's aphasics who were judged by speech therapists as exhibiting "labored speech" did display elongated segments. These results suggest that the perception of dysfluency in the speech of some Broca's aphasics may be based on increased frequency and length of pauses, not on elongation of speech segments.

In rare cases, the intonational disorder in anterior aphasia produces the impression of a newly acquired foreign accent (Pick, 1908; Monrad-Krohn, 1947; Whitaker, 1982; Graff-Radford et al., 1986). In a classic case described by Monrad-Krohn, a Norwegian woman sustained a schrapnel wound to the left anterior region during World War II and subsequently acquired a German accent, problematic in her town given the attitude toward the German occupation. In more recent work, acoustical studies have pinpointed some of the characteristics of foreign accent in other patients with anterior lesions, but not enough cases have been studied to indicate whether a particular neural site is responsible for such accent. It is possible that the newly acquired accent is epiphenomenal, an impression of listeners resulting from separable intonational deficits. More cases of acquired foreign accent need to be examined before a clear account of the accent can be provided.

In summary, the speech of Broca's aphasics is typified by elongation of speech segments and pauses as well as some abnormalities in F_0. The general characterization of Broca's speech as *dysfluent*, made initially on the basis of clinical observation, holds true with more detailed acoustical study. On the other hand, acoustical analyses have revealed that some rudimentary features of normal F_0 production remain intact in Broca's speech despite long interword pauses.

WERNICKE'S APHASIA

In marked contrast to the utterances of Broca's aphasics, Wernicke's speech is quite fluent and gives the appearance of nearly normal prosody in clinical evaluation. Duchan, Stengel, and Oliva (1980), for example, remark that intonation contours of a jargon aphasic are generally appropriate, respecting syntactic boundaries and other structural aspects of sentences. Lecours and Rouillon (1976) have noted, however, that intonation is exaggerated in the speech of some Wernicke's aphasics, and a recent acoustical study of such patients supports this observation (Cooper, Danly, & Hamby, 1979).

A careful analysis of Wernicke's speech reveals other systematic irregularities that provide information relevant to the conceptual view previously outlined. We shall consider two studies that combine acoustical measures of Wernicke's speech with some consideration of the unique characteristics of the disorder.

In one study, hesitation pauses in the spontaneous interview speech of a single patient were analyzed to determine whether any relation existed between the amount of pausing and the presence of immediately following neologisms or paraphasias (Butterworth, 1979). The results showed that the aphasic produced significantly longer pauses preceding neologisms than preceding paraphasias. In addition, the appearance of a hesitation was more likely preceding neologisms, with about one-half of the neologisms being preceded by a pause, compared with only about one-fourth of the verbal paraphasias. Butterworth hypothesized that the speaker's neologisms represent an adaptation to a failure of lexical search, which presumably takes place during at least part of the pause interval—the key assumption here being that hesitation pausing represents an interval of silence during which the speaker is engaged in word-finding activity, and correspondingly that neologistic forms are not simply inserted by the speaker because the normal constraints on word formation are disinhibited.

A detailed analysis of the pause durations revealed a systematic difference in the durations associated with "pure" neologisms—bearing no phonological relation to either the target word or to an adjacent word in the utterance—and neologisms that did bear some such phonological relation. The pause durations for the "pure" neologisms were about twice as long as average, suggesting that these neologisms were produced by a special device that generates a stereotypical nonsense form when lexical search is aborted. In addition, the pauses preceding phonologically related neologisms were about twice as long as pauses preceding verbal paraphasias. Butterworth's claim that neologisms are often produced by a special device is supported by evidence from other investigators who have reported that some individual patients' neologisms often have a stereotypical phonological form (e.g., Green, 1969; Lhermitte et al., 1973; Buckingham, 1974; Duchan et al., 1980, and references therein). Unlike Butterworth, however, Duchan and colleagues report informally an absence of long pauses before neologisms in the speech of one jargon aphasic, suggesting that this patient either does not require pausing for lexical search at the locations eventually occupied by neologisms (perhaps lexical search for the key word is planned ahead of time) or that neologisms for this speaker do not in fact represent a replacement for aborted lexical search.

The locations of neologisms within an utterance may eventually provide another peg of support for the view that these forms reflect a failure of lexical search. Green (1969) observed that neologisms generally appear in the predicate rather than the subject noun phrase of Wernicke's speech. This finding suggests that the patient might adopt a strategy of withholding speech until the lexical and phonological representation of the subject NP is programmed, with the predicate being unspecified in large part before speech is initiated. According to this view, neologisms appear primarily within the predicate because the speaker incurs the most difficulty with lexical search in this region. Alternatively, the finding that neologisms appear more prevalently in the predicate may simply be due to the fact that more words generally appear in the predicate, rendering more individual opportunities for lexical search difficulty. Both Green (1969) and Butterworth (1979) report that the bulk of neologisms replace target nouns, but more nouns typically appear in the predicate of a sentence than in the subject, and future work must be conducted to unravel the alternative accounts of this predicate effect.

The relationship between pausing and neologisms observed by Butterworth and others also appears to distinguish the word-finding difficulty of Wernicke's aphasics from that of anomics. As noted by Buckingham (1979), anomic patients typically exhibit hesitation pauses in the absence of neologisms when they incur word-finding difficulty, whereas Wernicke's aphasics are more likely to exhibit neologisms immediately following hesitation pauses. One question that remains, however, is whether the neologisms prevalent in Wernicke's speech reflect the output of a special device utilized as part of a clever strategy for camouflaging difficulty with word-finding, as Butterworth suggests, or whether these neologisms represent a natural consequence of partial retrieval of lexical information, including a few semantic and phonological features that are combined to form a neologistic output (e.g., Marshall, 1979). The stereotypical form of many neologisms for an individual patient does seem to implicate a special generation device.

Recently, a general acoustical analysis of speech prosody in Wernicke's speech has been undertaken to determine whether such patients exhibit subtle but systematic prosodic deficits that typically go undetected during informal clinical observation (Cooper, et al., 1979). Salient aspects of fundamental frequency contours in sentence contexts were examined, including the form of F_O declination and the first peak value of F_O in relatively long versus short sentences. As noted earlier, for normal subjects, the form of F_O declination for successive peaks in a single main-clause sentence can be captured by an abstract mathematical rule. Given the first and last peak values and their times of occurrence, the rule can adequately predict the F_O values of intermediate peaks in the utterance, largely invariant across a wide variety of variables such as speaker sex, speaking rate, sentence length, and others (Cooper & Sorensen, 1981). By examining the detailed form of declination for Wernicke's speech in the same sentence contexts, it was possible to determine whether their speech adhered to this mathematical formulation and whether their declination was perturbed in any way by the presence of paraphasias or neologisms.

In addition to this issue, the F_O values of the first peak in long versus short utterances were examined, as in the study of Broca's speech, to determine whether Wernicke's exhibit long-range planning in their speech prosody. Recall that, in normal speech, the first peak in a longer single-clause sentence is higher in F_O than is the first peak in a shorter sentence.

The results of the study indicated that Wernicke's speech does exhibit systematic departures from the oral reading of normals. Of 5 patients tested, 4 regularly exhibited some form of F_O declination, but none of these patients adhered to the mathematical formulation of declination in a normal fashion. The patients generally started their first peak in F_O higher than normal for both long and short sentences. The peak values for this first peak did not differ significantly in the long versus short sentences, however, indicating another departure from normal speech. Like Broca's aphasics, Wernicke's patients do not seem to take into account the overall length of the target utterance in programming their first F_O peak, suggesting a deficit in long-range planning capability. Since their values for the first peak were higher than normal for all sentences, this possible failure did not lead to a restriction in the range of F_O declination in long sentences, however.

Perhaps the most interesting finding of this study was that the form of the aphasic's declination was relatively unperturbed by the presence of paraphasias or neologisms. This result was most apparent for a patient who produced literal paraphasias for approximately half of the key words spoken correctly. The similarity of the declination functions for correct and paraphasic output for this and other patients suggests that the programming of F_O declination proceeds in a manner that is relatively independent of proper phoneme selection.

In addition to these findings, the acoustical analysis revealed other abnormalities in the oral reading of Wernicke's patients. Although the sentences used in the study involved simple syntactic structures and relatively high frequency words, the speech of the patients was, on average, almost twice as slow as normal, primarily due to an increase in hesitation pauses just prior to content words. This finding suggests that Wernicke's speakers are not really very "fluent" in a demanding reading situation and that their apparent fluency in spontaneous speech derives from their ability to cover up problems of lexical retrieval by producing neologisms and circumlocutions, as discussed earlier in relation to studies of pausing (e.g., Butterworth, 1979). In addition, Wernicke's speech displayed larger than normal peak-to-valley fluctuations in F_O, indicating that their fundamental frequency is often more contrastive than normal, which supports the observation of Lecours and Rouillon (1976).

In conclusion, while the speech of Wernicke's aphasics is far more fluent than that of Broca's, it does exhibit prosodic abnormalities. Regarding speech timing, hesitation pauses often precede neologisms, and it appears that these two features in conjunction represent difficulty in word-finding. The finding that neologisms are likely to follow hesitation pauses allows one to infer that neologisms represent a default output when lexical search fails. It seems quite possible that these neologisms are generated by a special device and serve to camouflage the speaker's failure to retrieve target words.

The fundamental frequency of Wernicke's speech shows more of a tendency toward declination of peaks than does Broca's speech, although the precise programming of declination is not equivalent to normal speech. In addition, Wernicke's aphasics show the same deficit in long-term planning as Broca's for programming the first F_O peak of an utterance with respect to the overall length of the utterance. Despite these deficits, Wernicke's programming of F_O seems largely unperturbed by the presence of literal paraphasias and neologisms, suggesting that the operations involved in programming F_O are, for the most part, independent from those that select phonemes.

RIGHT-HEMISPHERE LESIONS

Comparison of patients with unilateral damage to either the left or right cerebral hemispheres provides information about the extent to which intonational programming is conducted unilaterally. While unilateral damage to the right cerebral hemisphere generally spares the language faculty in right-handed patients, such damage produces certain abnormalities in the intonational aspects of speech production and comprehension (Dordain, Degos, & Dordain, 1971; Tucker, Watson, & Heilman, 1977; Ross & Mesulam, 1979; Weintraub, Mesulam, & Kramer, 1981; Cooper et al., 1984; Shapiro & Danly, 1985). Intonational deficits are particularly apparent for these patients during affective speech, but deficits have been noted for linguistic intonational features as well. For example, Shapiro and Danly (1985) found that F_O rises associated with yes–no questions are greatly attenuated in patients with right-anterior or central lesions, and Cooper and colleagues (1984) found that the effects of clause and utterance length on intonation are also attenuated in patients with right hemisphere lesions. Results such as these are important since the loss of affective intonation alone would not necessarily imply that the right hemisphere is directly involved in intonational processing. Instead, such loss could occur as a secondary consequence of right hemisphere involvement in processing emotional characteristics (e.g., Heilman, Scholes, & Watson, 1975; Tucker, Watson, & Heilman, 1977; Wapner, Hamby, & Gardner, 1981), which, in turn, are known to influence speech intonation (e.g., Williams & Stevens, 1972; Cosmides, 1983). Intonational deficits found during nonemotional speech, however, imply an intrinsic disorder of the processing mechanisms responsible for intonational characteristics.

While right-hemisphere patients apparently do exhibit linguistic intonational deficits, these deficits may be less severe for right- than for left-hemisphere patients. For example, Cooper and colleagues (1984) observed that intonational deficits related to clause and utterance length were generally more pronounced for patients with left rather than right-hemisphere lesions. These findings dovetail with a study of Norwegian tone by Ryalls and Reinvang (1986), in which relatively greater impairments were observed for patients with left-hemisphere damage (See also Behrens, Chapter 5, for other evidence of retained prosody in right-hemisphere patients).

A variable that needs to be examined in more detail is precise localization and extent of lesion within the right hemisphere. Recent studies suggest that damage to different portions of the right hemisphere may be accompanied by different sorts of deficits in speakers' productions of F_O (Dordain et al., 1971; Cooper et al., 1984; Shapiro & Danly, 1985). However, the picture involving intonation-lesion associations with these patients is less clear than is the picture involving such associations with patients sustaining left-hemisphere damage. For example, in a recent study of 11 right-hemisphere patients, including 3 anteriors, 3 centrals, and 5 posteriors, Shapiro and Danly (1985) found that anterior and central subgroups were amelodic, exhibiting less pitch variation and a restricted intonational range, compared to control subjects and posterior patients, who appeared somewhat hypermelodic. However, the authors indicate that the patient groups included in their study were not homogeneous with respect to intonational contours. That is, not all posterior patients displayed hypermelodicity, and not all anterior-centrals were intonationally flat. In addition, Cooper et al. (1984) found essentially normal F_O contours in their anterior-central patients.

The inconsistency of these results may be related to differences among patients in premorbid speech characteristics or to speech-influencing disorder complications such as depression. In addition, Ryalls (1986b) and Colsher, Cooper, & Graff-Radford (1986a) point out that mean and variance of nontransformed F_O measures tend to be correlated, suggesting that mean pitch ought to be taken into account in studies of aprosody and hypermelodicity. For example, Colsher and colleagues note that the anterior patients studied by Shapiro and Danly (1985) exhibit relatively low mean F_O values as well as low F_O variability, and that when the variability measures are normalized for mean F_O, the anteriors actually exhibit somewhat higher variability than the normals. Colsher and colleagues further explored this issue using new speech samples from two right-hemisphere patients and three control speakers. They found that the right hemisphere patients exhibited higher mean F_O and greater F_O variability than did the control subjects. However, when standard deviations were normalized for mean F_O, the control patients exhibited the greatest variability.

Another recent study by Colsher and colleagues (1986b) indicates that time post-onset should also be considered when assessing intonation in right-hemisphere patients. They found that patients tested soon after stroke tended to produce amelodic, compressed F_O contours, whereas patients tested 6 months post-onset tended to produce hypermelodic or normal F_O contours. These findings, while preliminary, suggest that some of the apparent discrepancies between amelodic and hypermelodic intonation reported in the literature might be attributable to the variable of time post-onset, a variable that needs to be considered more precisely in future work. Thus it seems premature to draw conclusions regarding the extent to which the basic anterior–posterior distinction among lesions provides the best single dichotomy in distinguishing intonational deficits associated with lesions of the right hemisphere in a manner homologous to lesions of the left hemisphere (cf. Ross & Mesulam, 1979; Ross, 1981).

Although the studies reviewed here indicate that the right hemisphere ordinarily contributes to the processing of intonational information, studies of split-brain patients suggest that the disconnected right hemisphere does not as a rule possess the capacity for speech production (see Gazzaniga, 1983, for a review). Thus, it might be assumed that any intonational information processed in the right hemisphere must in some way be transferred to the left-hemisphere speech centers during speech production. Several researchers have suggested that this integrative function most likely occurs via the corpus callosum (e.g., Ross et al., 1981; Speedie, Coslett, & Heilman, 1984). Indeed, evidence from a case of callosal disconnection (Watson & Heilman, 1983) indicates an inability to repeat affective tone properly. In addition, a recent acoustic investigation of intonation following callosal damage indicates deficits for linguistic as well as affective prosodic distinctions immediately following surgery (Klouda et al., 1986). In this study, the patient was tested at 4, 12, and 24 weeks postsurgery, and, interestingly, showed considerable improvement with respect to both affective and linguistic F_O distinctions as a function of time. Furthermore, these improvements in speech production were accompanied by improvements in the perceptual judgment of her intended tone by normal listeners. Such improvement may imply that, while the right hemisphere generally contributes to F_O programming, following callosal damage, such programming can later be performed by the left hemisphere. This hypothesis is supported by evidence that some right-brain-damaged patients also exhibit more normal F_O patterns when tested at 6 months rather than immediately post-stroke (Colsher et al., 1986b).

FUTURE DIRECTIONS

In the case of aphasia and related disorders, it is much easier to contemplate the kinds of studies that one would like to see done than to get on with the business of actually conducting them. Accordingly, this section will at best provide modest guidelines, ultimately of value only if they are supplanted by the kinds of empirical studies they suggest. To date, the information on intonation and brain damage is quite sketchy and should be considered preliminary in all major respects.

If future work is to attain a definitive status, some major improvements need to be made in terms of testing larger sample sizes, controlling more tightly such factors as age, educational level, medication, and time post-onset, and providing additional controls to ferret out complicating emotional or other disorders, among others. To cite one example, it would be helpful to have Beck depression scores on all patients, to be correlated with intonational performance so that any depressive component of intonational impairment can be distinguished from a neurological one. In addition, nonlinguistic production tasks such as humming might be included in testing to determine whether intonational deficits are distinctively linguistic. The issue of larger sample sizes is probably the most serious and is needed if neuroimaging techniques are to be successfully utilized in conjunction with behavioral testing to adequately characterize many brain-behavior relations. The issues that occupy future researchers will probably include many of the ones examined thus far, including modularity and localization. However, advances in behavioral testing should lead to the formulation of new issues as well, particularly ones emphasizing the processing mechanisms involved in the programming of intonation, including both psychological and physiological aspects.

ACKNOWLEDGMENTS

Preparation of this chapter was supported by NIH Grant NS 20071. Portions of this chapter have been adapted from material originally contained in a chapter by W.E. Cooper and E.B. Zurif, "Aphasia: Information-processing in language production and reception," appearing in B. Butterworth (ed.) *Language Production*: Vol. 2. London: Academic Press, 1983.

REFERENCES

Blumstein, S.E., & Milberg, W. (1983). Automatic and controlled processing in speech/language deficits in aphasia (Paper presented at the Academy of Aphasia, Minneapolis).

Branigan, G. (1976a). Sequences of single words on structural units (Paper presented at the Eighth Annual Child Language Research Forum, Stanford University).

Branigan, G. (1976b). Organizational constraints during the one-word period (Paper presented at the First Annual Boston University Conference on Language Development).

Breckenridge, J. (1977). Declination as a phonological process. *Bell Laboratories Technological Memo*, Murray Hill, NJ: Bell Laboratories.

Broca, P. (1861). Remarques sur le siege de la faculte du langage articule, suives d'une observation d'aphemie. *Bulletin de la Societe de Anatomie de Paris*, 330–357.

Buckingham, H.W., Jr. (1979) Linguistic aspects of lexical retrieval disturbances in the posterior fluent aphasias. In H. Whitaker & H.A. Whitaker (Eds.), *Studies in neurolinguistics, Vol. 4*. New York: Academic Press.

Buckingham, H.W. Jr. (1974). A neurolinguistic description of neologistic jargon aphasia (Doctoral dissertation, University of Rochester).

Butterworth, B. (1979). Hesitation and the production of verbal paraphasias and neologisms in jargon aphasia. *Brain and Language, 8*, 133–161.

Colsher, P.L., Cooper, W.E., & Graff-Radford, N.R. (1986a). Intonational variability in the speech of right-hemisphere damaged patients. *Brain and Language*, in press.

Colsher, P.L., Cooper, W.E., & Graff-Radford, N.R. (1986b). Intonational characteristics of right-hemisphere damaged, patients' speech and its perception by normal listeners (submitted for publication).

Cooper, W.E., Danly, M., & Hamby, S. (1979). Fundamental frequency F_0 attributes in the speech of Wernicke's aphasics. In J.J. Wolf and D.H. Klatt (Eds.), *Speech Communication Papers Presented at the 97th Meeting of the Acoustical Society of America*, New York: Acoustical Society of America.

Cooper, W.E., Eady, S.J., & Mueller, P.R. (1985). Acoustical aspects of contrastive stress in question-answer contexts. *Journal of the Acoustical Society of America, 77*, 2142–2156.

Cooper, W.E., & Ehrlich, S.F. (1981). Planning speech: Studies in choice reaction time. In A. Baddeley & J. Long (Eds.), *Attention and Performance IX*. Hillsdale, NJ: Lawrence Erlbaum Associates.

Cooper, W.E., Soares, C., Nicol, J., Michelow, D., & Goloskie, S. (1984). Clausal intonation after unilateral brain damage. *Language and Speech, 27*, 17–24.

Cooper, W.E., & Sorensen, J.M. (1977). Fundamental frequency contours at syntactic boundaries. *Journal of the Acoustical Society of America, 62*, 682–692.

Cooper, W.E., & Sorensen, J.M. (1981). *Fundamental frequency in sentence production*. New York: Springer-Verlag.

Cosmides, L. (1983). Invariances in the acoustic expression of emotion during speech. *Journal of Experimental Psychology: Human Perception and Performance. 9*, 864–881.

Danly, M., Cooper, W.E., & Shapiro, B. (1983). Fundamental frequency, language processing, and linguistic structure in Wernicke's aphasia. *Brain and Language, 19*, 1–24.

Danly, M., de Villiers, J.G., & Cooper, W.E. (1979). Control of speech prosody in Broca's aphasia. In J.J. Wolf & D.H. Klatt (Eds.), *Speech Communication Papers Presented at the 97th Meeting of the Acoustical Society of America*, New York: Acoustical Society of America.

Danly, M., & Shapiro, B. (1982). Speech prosody in Broca's aphasia. *Brain and Language, 16*, 171–190.

Demeurisse, G., Demol, 0., Robaye, E., Coekaerts, M.-J., de Beuckelaer, R., & Derouck, M. (1979). Quantitative evaluation of aphasia resulting from a cerebral vascular accident. *Neuropsychologia, 17,* 55–65.

Dordain, M., Degos, J.D., & Dordain, G. (1971). Troubles de la voix dans les hemiplegies gauches. *Revue de Laryngologie, 92,* 178–188.

Duchan, J.F., Stengel, M.L., & Oliva, J. (1980). A dynamic phonological model derived from the intonational analysis of a jargon aphasic patient. *Brain and Language, 9,* 289–297.

Gazzaniga, M.S. (1983). Right hemisphere language following brain bisection: A 20-year perspective. *American Psychologist, 38,* 525–541.

Goodglass, H., Fodor, I., & Schulhoff, C. (1967). Prosodic factors in grammar-evidence from aphasia. *Journal of Speech and Hearing Research, 10,* 5–20.

Goodglass, H., & Kaplan, E. (1972). *The assessment of aphasia and related disorders.* Philadelphia: Lea and Febiger.

Graff-Radford, N.R., Cooper, W.E., Colsher, P.L., & Damasio, A.R. (1986). An unlearned foreign "accent" in a patient with aphasia. *Brain and Language, 28* 86–94.

Green, E. (1969). Phonological and grammatical aspects of jargon in an aphasic patient. *Language and Speech, 12,* 103–118.

Heilman, K.M., Scholes, R., & Watson, R.T. (1975). Auditory affective agnosia: Disturbed comprehension of affective speech. *Journal of Neurology, Neurosurgery, and Psychiatry, 38,* 69–72.

Klatt, D.H. (1975). Vowel lengthening is syntactically determined in a connected discourse. *Journal of Phonetics, 3,* 129–140.

Klouda, G.V., Robin, D.A., Graff-Radford, N.R., & Cooper, W.E. (1986). Intonational impairment following naturally occurring callosal disconnection (Under review).

Kreindler, A., Mihailescu, L., & Fradis, A. (1980). Speech fluency in aphasics. *Brain and Language, 9,* 199–205.

Lea, W.A. (1973). Segmental and suprasegmental influences on fundamental frequency contours. In L.M. Hyman (Ed.), *Consonant types and tone.* Los Angeles: USC Press, pp. 15–70.

Lecours, A.R., & Rouillon, F. (1976). Neurolinguistic analysis of jargonaphasia and jargonagraphia. In H. Whitaker & H.A. Whitaker (Eds.), *Studies in Neurolinguistics* (Vol. 2). New York and London: Academic Press.

Lhermitte, F., Lecours, A.R., Ducarne, B., & Escourolle, R. (1973). Unexpected anatomical findings in a case of fluent jargon aphasia. *Cortex, 9,* 433–446.

Lieberman, P. (1965). On the acoustic basis of the perception of intonation by linguists. *Word, 21,* 40–54.

Lyberg, B. (1979). Final lengthening–partly a consequence of restrictions on the speed of fundamental frequency change? *Journal of Phonetics, 7,* 187–196.

Marshall, J.C. (1979). Disorder in the expression of language. In J. Morton & J.C. Marshall (Eds.), *Psycholinguistics.* Cambridge, MA: MIT Press.

Martin, J.G. (1970). On judging pauses in spontaneous speech. *Journal of Verbal Learning and Verbal Behavior, 9,* 75–78.

Monrad-Krohn, G.H. (1947). Dysprosody or altered "melody of language." *Brain, 70,* 405–415.

Pick, A. (1931). *Aphasia.* (Translated by Jason W. Brown, London: Charles Thomas, 1973).

Ross, E.D. (1981). The aprosodias: Functional-anatomic organization of the affective components of language in the right hemisphere. *Archives of Neurology, 38,* 561–569.

Ross, E.D., Harney, J.H., deLacoste-Utamsing, C., & Purdy, P. (1981). How the brain integrates affective and propositional language into a unified behavioral function. *Archives of Neurology, 38,* 745–748.

Ross, E.D., & Mesulam, M. (1979). Dominant language functions of the right hemisphere? Prosody or emotional gesturing. *Archives of Neurology, 35,* 144–148.

Ryalls, J.H. (1982). Intonation in Broca's Aphasia. *Neuropsychologia, 20,* 355–360.

Ryalls, J.H. (1986a). An acoustic study of vowel production in aphasia. *Brain and Language, 29,* 48–67.

Ryalls, J.H. (1986b). What constitutes a primary disturbance of speech prosody?: A reply to Shapiro and Danly. *Brain and Language, 29,* 183–187.

Ryalls, J.H., and Reinvang, I. (1986). Functional lateralization of linguistic tones: Acoustic evidence from Norwegian. *Language and Speech, 29,* 389–398.

Selkirk, E.0. (1984). *Phonology and syntax: The relation between sound and structure.* Cambridge, MA: MIT Press.

Shapiro, B., & Danly, M. (1985). The role of the right hemisphere in the control of speech prosody in propositional and affective contexts. *Brain and Language, 25,* 19–36.

Speedie, L.J., Coslett, H.B., & Heilman, K.M. (1984). Repetition of affective prosody in mixed transcortical aphasia. *Archives of Neurology, 41,* 268–270.

Tucker, D.M., Watson, R.T., & Heilman, K.M. (1977). Discrimination and evocation of affectively intoned speech in patients with right parietal disease. *Neurology, 27,* 947–950.

Wagenaar, E., Snow, C., & Prins, R. (1975). Spontaneous speech of aphasic patients: A psycholinguistic analysis. *Brain and Language, 2,* 281–303.

Wapner, W., Hamby, S., & Gardner, H. (1981). The role of the right hemisphere in the apprehension of complex linguistic material. *Brain and Language, 14,* 15–33.

Watson, R.T., & Heilman, K.M. (1983). Callosal Apraxia. *Brain, 106,* 391–403.

Weintraub, S., Mesulam, M., & Kramer, L. (1981). Disturbances in prosody: A right hemisphere contribution to language. *Archives of Neurology, 38,* 742–744.

Whitaker, H. (1982). Levels of impairment in disorders of speech. In R.N. Malatesha & L.C. Hartlage (Eds.). *Neuropsychology and cognition* (Vol. 1). The Hague: Nijhoff (Nato Advanced Study Institutes Series D, No.9).

Williams, C.E., & Stevens, K.N. (1972). Emotions and speech: Some acoustical correlates. *Journal of the Acoustical Society of America, 52,* 1238–1250.

Williams, S.E., & Seaver, E.J. (1986). A comparison of speech sound durations in three syndromes of aphasia. *Brain and Language, 29,* 171–182.

P A R T   II

New Data

The Role of the Right Hemisphere in the Production of Linguistic Prosody: An Acoustic Investigation

Susan J. Behrens

A recent question in the field of neurolinguistics is whether a general prosodic disturbance, one encompassing both emotional and linguistic domains, can be associated with right-hemisphere damage (RHD) (Weintraub, Mesulam & Kramer, 1981; Shapiro & Danly, 1985). A common set of acoustic parameters (amplitude, duration, and fundamental frequency (F_O)) underlies both domains of prosody (Lieberman & Michaels, 1962; Monrad-Krohn, 1947; 1963; Williams & Stevens, 1972), thereby suggesting to many researchers that the emotional dysprosody reported in RHD patients (e.g., Heilman, Scholes, & Watson, 1975; Ross, 1981) may be a consequence of a general problem in the control of these acoustic correlates.

Several studies have tested this theory by concentrating on the integrity of linguistic prosody in RHD speakers. Investigations into the ability of RHD patients to produce linguistic prosody have examined prosody at the sentence level (Cooper et al., 1984; Shapiro & Danly, 1985; Behrens, 1986) and at the word level (Weintraub et al., 1981; Behrens, in press; Emmorey, 1987). Word stress in English serves several functions, one being to signal the distinction between such phrases as *lighthouse* (a compound noun) and *light house* (adjective and noun, or noun phrase (NP)). This function is termed phonemic stress, and the ability of RHD speakers to produce phonemic stress will be the focus of this chapter.

Studies focusing on the comprehension of semantic distinctions signalled by phonemic stress have been administered to normal, left-hemisphere damaged (LHD) aphasic, and RHD subjects, and the overall results present a mixed view of a cerebral dominance for the processing of phonemic stress. Behrens (1985) found that in a dichotic listening task, normal subjects asked to identify stress placement on such pairs as *Redcoat* and *red coat* displayed right-ear advantages, but a new group of subjects demonstrated left-ear advantages when the same stimuli were low-pass filtered to obliterate the phonetic structure. These data suggest that stress fulfilling a linguistic function engages a left hemisphere mechanism, while prosody in a nonphonetic context may entail a superior right-hemisphere processor.

Baum et al. (1982) also report evidence of left hemisphere dominance for linguistic stress. They found that LHD Broca's aphasic patients performed significantly worse than normal controls in distinguishing between compound nouns and NP items. The authors concluded that the aphasic patients may have a deficit in processing variations in the acoustic information that signals stress, thereby implying a left hemisphere mechanism for linguistic stress.

The results of Baum and colleagues are in contradiction to those of Blumstein and Goodglass (1972), who also studied the ability of LHD aphasic patients to distinguish between phrases differing only by location of primary stress. When presented with one member of a stress pair and instructed to point to the appropriate illustration of the meaning, accuracy was high. Although left-hemisphere damage did not affect the ability to perceive phonemic differences signalled by stress placement, it is still possible that the perception of stress contrasts is a left-hemisphere ability.

Exploring RHD patients' ability to process phonemic stress, using the same stimuli as Blumstein and Goodglass (1972), Weintraub and colleagues (1981) found that the semantic distinctions signalled by the stress contrasts proved more difficult for these patients to make than for control subjects with no brain damage. Weintraub and colleagues conclude that, taken together with reports of emotional dysprosody in RHD groups, their data support a view of general prosodic disruption in this patient population. Weintraub and colleagues, however, failed to conduct acoustic analyses on their subjects' productions; their conclusions are instead based on the investigators' own judgments of prosodic prominence.

Emmorey (1987) did carry out acoustical analysis, examining subjects' use of duration and F_O to distinguish between bisyllabic stress pairs in the speech of LHD aphasic patients, RHD speakers, and normal controls. Each speaker's productions were analyzed separately to determine how each individual signalled the semantic distinction: through duration changes from the compound noun to the NP form in either syllable of the phrases, by a greater fluctuation in F_O from syllable one to two in one phrase compared to its stress counterpart, or by a greater pause between syllables in one type of phrase.

A majority of normal control speakers utilized both duration and F_O to convey one meaning over the other.[1] Nonfluent aphasics, on the other

---

[1]In reporting duration results, Emmorey fails to distinguish between measures taken of the syllable and intersyllabic pause measures.

hand, failed to make use of F_O change at all and only half the speakers conveyed a meaning difference through a distinction in duration. Fifty percent of fluent aphasic subjects altered both duration and F_O in a comparison of their stress pairs. RHD speakers, though, most resembled the normals—all but one displaying changes in duration and F_O from one phrase to its stress counterpart. A post-test investigating the perceptual saliency of all speakers' stress placement showed a significant correlation between acoustically robust stress changes (as indicated by duration and F_O measures) and perceptually strong stress placement. Thus, Emmorey concluded that RHD was associated with an intact ability to produce stress contrasts.

The goal of Emmorey's study was similar to that of Behrens (in press), in which the ability to produce phonemic stress and emphatic stress was explored in RHD speakers. Acoustic analysis conducted by Behrens considered not only duration and F_O properties associated with stress, but amplitude as well. In addition, more natural speech was elicited through use of story-completion tasks, in contrast to a reading task employed in Emmorey. This is an important methodological concern, for past studies have shown acoustic differences to be apparent between utterances obtained through read or imitative speech and spontaneous speech samples (Umeda, 1982; Lieberman et al., 1985), and using more natural speech samples guarantees a clearer picture of production abilities.

A report of data in Behrens (in press), together with those of Emmorey, will offer a more controlled view of right hemisphere ability to produce phonemic stress, one derived from acoustic measures and statistical testing rather than subjective judgments. A brief discussion of previous acoustic analyses of word stress, obtained from normal speakers, will first be presented to better delineate the acoustic attributes of linguistic stress.

ACOUSTIC CORRELATES OF LINGUISTIC PROSODY

Placement of primary stress in English manifests itself in various acoustic alterations of the stressed syllable compared to an unstressed counterpart (cf., Fry, 1955, and Lieberman, 1960). Further, the effects of stress placement on vowels appear to be more robust than on consonants (Oller, 1973; Klatt, 1976). Klatt (1976), concentrating on duration cues, noted that the vowel of a stressed syllable is longer than that of an unstressed syllable. This difference is most extreme in phrase-final syllables. McClean and Tiffany (1973) report similar findings. Segments occurring in various lexical positions, then (e.g., *initially, finally*), may acquire the acoustic characteristics intrinsic to those positions, thus interacting with the effects of stress.

McClean and Tiffany (1973) examined stressed and unstressed vowels in the nonsense phrases [sá sa] and [sa sá]. They found that, irrespective of position, the stressed syllable was greater in amplitude and higher in F_O, compared to the unstressed syllable. Considering syllable position, independent of stress placement, McClean and Tiffany found initial syllables to be higher in F_O than final syllables. Further, when initial syllables were unstressed, they still displayed higher F_O compared to stressed final syllables. For the stress pattern in [sá sa], the researchers found a greater F_O difference from first to second syllable than in [sa sá]. No effect of syllable position with regard to amplitude was obtained, however.

In order to obtain measures of acoustic correlates to word stress without confounding syllable position, and to normalize for speakers' inconsistency in loudness or rate, a measure which captures the relative acoustic nature from utterance to utterance must be employed. Lieberman (1960) analyzed noun–verb stress pairs such as reb'el (a revolutionary) and rebel' (the action of fighting against). Extracting measures of F_O, amplitude, and duration for each syllable of the test words, he calculated proportional measures for each acoustic parameter in two ways: (1) by dividing the stressed syllable by the unstressed syllable for a single utterance; and (2) by dividing the stressed syllable of one word by the unstressed syllable of its counterpart. In this way, the *relative* change from syllable to syllable for each word could be quantified and compared to the same word displaying the alternate stress pattern.

Within word comparisons (comparison type [1]), Lieberman found stressed syllables to be higher in F_O for 90% of the utterances analyzed, higher in amplitude 87% of the time, and longer 66% of the time. For the second type of comparison, across words, amplitude was found to constitute a more reliable measure of stress: the stressed syllable was higher in amplitude 90% of the time, with a greater F_O value for 72% of the cases.

Although Lieberman found a certain degree of speaker variation in the combinations of stress cues used to signal nouns from verbs, consistent patterns emerged: no stressed syllable was ever lower in both amplitude and F_O compared to an unstressed comparison. In addition, if amplitude proved a weak cue to stress in a production, duration was found to be greater in the stressed syllable. A tradeoff exists, then, between these three parameters, allowing for individual variation.

Similar findings are reported by Emmorey (1987). Duration measures for each syllable position (e.g., *initial, final*) were compared across stress patterns to determine which portion of the phrase was most utilized in signaling the meaning difference, or in other words, which word showed the greatest acoustic change with a stress shift. The difference in F_O values across syllables for each phrase was also calculated, and this difference was compared for the two types of phrases. Emmorey found a range of acoustic correlates used by her speakers to distinguish one meaning from another.

Although phonetically similar segments were compared, e.g., *red* compared in the compound proper noun *Redcoat* and in the noun phrase *red coat*, certain information was lost by Emmorey's failure to consider relative acoustic properties within each phrase. Confounding factors such as inconsistent speaker intensity or rate might have manifested themselves in acoustic changes that were independent of stress placement. For example, both syllables of the NP items were found to be longer than both syllables of the compound noun stimuli. The relative duration from syllable-to-syllable (e.g., *red* compared to *coat*) may not have differed between the two phrase types, however, with the first syllable, for example, always two-thirds the length of the second syllable. Further, when Emmorey did compare syllables within an utterance, as she did for F_O, she computed the *absolute* difference from syllable to syllable rather than a relative value. This also is misleading, for it again says nothing of the proportionate values between syllables in phrases differing only by stress.

The present study, in contrast, adopted Lieberman's analysis technique of comparing ratios to quantify the acoustic nature of an utterance and comparing it to that same utterance with the alternate stress placement.

METHODS

Subjects

Subjects included 8 right-handed male speakers of American English who had suffered unilateral right hemisphere cerebrovascular accidents. The mean subject age was 62 years, and mean time postinfarct was 20 months. CAT scan information was not available for all patients, but for 2 RHD patients, lesions were localized as parietal, for 1 patient as frontal, and for 2 patients as injuries encompassing both the frontal and parietal lobes. A complete description and etiology of available lesion information for each patient may be obtained from Behrens (in press). All RHD speakers were patients at either the Boston or Providence V.A. Medical Center.[2] A group of 7 nonneurological male speakers comprised the control group. Mean age for the control group was 31 years.

Stimuli and Procedure

To obtain more natural speech samples from subjects, short scenarios were employed that required completion of a final target phrase. Each scenario corresponded to a picture of the target phrase, which was presented to the subject simultaneous with the scenarios. Pictures used in this task were a subset of those used by Blumstein and Goodglass (1972) and Baum and colleagues (1982). A tape recorder was used to record all responses

---

[2]A prescreening procedure ensured that all patients were capable of producing syllabic stress in general. Unambiguous polysyllabic words were read by these patients, and phonetically trained listeners determined that stress placement for all speakers was within normal limits.

of the subjects. The recorded responses were analyzed in two ways: First, acoustic measures were obtained to examine the types of cues used by subjects to signal stress placement. Measures were obtained of the duration (in ms) of the full vowel of each syllable, the amplitude (in dB) of each syllable, an intersyllabic pause measure, and the F_O of each syllable's vowel. The perceptual saliency of these emergining cues was also investigated to determine the perceptual consequences of varying combinations of acoustic correlates. The perceptual saliency of each utterance was determined by presentation of all tokens to three phonetically trained listeners who determined the placement of primary stress.

ACOUSTIC AND PERCEPTUAL ANALYSES:
RESULTS AND DISCUSSION

Results for Normal Speakers

Table 5-1 presents the mean values for the control group, by syllable position and stress pattern, for all parameters. These values indicate that, for amplitude, initial syllables are on average greater compared to final syllables. An interaction of syllable position and stress is evident, though, in that the syllable-to-syllable amplitude difference is of a greater magnitude for the compound noun tokens compared to the NP items. Duration values also are on average greater for one syllable position, the final syllable, but the syllable-to-syllable difference is of a greater magnitude for the noun phrases. Initial syllables are also higher in F_O, irrespective of phrase type, with a greater F_O fall across syllables in the compound tokens. Finally, pause measures are greater in the NP items, as noted in previous studies (Bolinger & Gerstman, 1957; Emmorey, 1987).

Lieberman (1960) noted speaker-to-speaker variation in the combination of stress cues evident for his subjects. Item analyses were performed on each subject's productions in the present study to investigate the pattern of cues that might emerge. Separate statistical testing was conducted on each subject's productions for each measure. We are mainly interested in whether the acoustic manifestations of stress were a function of both syllable position and phrase type. A significant interaction, signalling that the acoustic patterns of the stimuli were a function of these two factors, thus were considered as indicating the presence of a stress cue for that parameter. Table 5-2 summarizes the results, indicating with a plus (+) sign where significant syllable by phrase-type interactions were obtained.

Subject variability can be observed, in that each subject makes use of a different combination of cues. Notice also that no speaker made use of all four cues and that two subjects appear to produce no stress correlates.

TABLE 5-1. Means of Stress Placement by Normal Subjects

S	1st Syll. Stress	2nd Syll. Unstress	1st Syll. Unstress	2nd Syll. Stress
Amplitude (in dB)	62	57	63	59
Duration (in ms)	104	116	129	156
F_o (in Hz)	102	86	104	93
Pause (in ms)	Compound Nouns 156*		194**	

*Compound nouns.
**Noun phrases.
Adapted from Behrens (in press).

The perceptual saliency of these combinations of cues, represented as mean percentages of correct identification by three listeners, are also listed in Table 5-2. To determine whether the two sets of data are correlated, statistical testing was conducted, which revealed a significant correlation between the number of cues present for a given subject and the corresponding perceptual scores. This correspondence is apparent, in that the two

TABLE 5-2. Summary of Stress Placement by Normal Subjects

S	Amplitude	Duration	F_o	Pause	Perception
1N	+	−	−	−	71%
2N	−	−	−	+	84
3N	+	−	−	+	87
4N	−	−	−	−	69
5N	−	+	+	+	94
6N	−	−	−	−	54
7N	−	−	+	+	X = 79

Plus (+) signs indicate significant interactions (p. < .05) between syllable position and stress pattern; minus (−) signs indicate nonsignificant interactions.
Adapted from Behrens (in press).

speakers failing to produce any stress cues also appear to have produced the least salient exemplars of phonemic stress, while stress placement in the production of speakers using two or more cues is identified most accurately by the three listeners.

Results for RHD Patients

Table 5-3 lists the group means for the RHD patients, by syllable and stress pattern. Unlike the normal data, final syllables are greater in amplitude compared to initial syllables, with a greater syllable-to-syllable change for the NP items. The groups appear more similar in the pattern of duration values, for which NP items on average show a greater degree of syllable to syllable change compared to compound nouns. Both subject groups also pattern similarly for F_O measures, with initial syllables higher compared to final syllables, and NP items displaying a greater F_O decrement across syllables. Intersyllabic pause values are also similar between groups, with NP items produced with greater pause duration.

Similar to the analyses of normal productions, statistical testing was conducted on each RHD patient's productions. Table 5-4 summarizes these results for the patients.

A majority of the patients appear to produce no stress cues, in marked contrast to the normal speakers. The two groups also appear to differ with respect to the corresponding identification scores, those for the RHD patients being lower (66%) than for the normal speakers (79%). There does not appear to be a high degree of correspondence between the two sets of data for the patients, especially noted in the results for S 4R. This speaker produced no statistically significant stress cues, yet the

TABLE 5-3. Means of Stress Placement by Patients

S	1st Syll. Stress	2nd Syll. Unstress	1st Syll. Unstress	2nd Syll. Stress
Amplitude (in dB)	55	56	54	57
Duration (in ms)	138	136	137	171
F_O (in Hz)	125	105	128	111
Pause (in ms)	Compound Nouns 151		172	

Adapted from Behrens (in press).

TABLE 5-4. Summary of Stress Placement by Patients

S	Amplitude	Duration	F_O	Pause	Perception
1R	—	—	—	—	47%
2R	—	—	—	—	56
3R	—	—	—	—	62
4R	—	—	—	—	80
5R	—	—	—	—	67
6R	+	—	—	—	72
7R	—	+	—	—	69
8R	—	—	+	—	73
					X = 66

Plus (+) signs indicate significant interactions (p. < .05) between syllable position and stress pattern; minus (−) signs indicate nonsignificant interactions.
Adapted from Behrens (in press).

corresponding perceptual score is quite high at 80%. This dissociation may reflect the emergence of partial cues not reaching statistical reliability or possible segmental cues that influenced listener judgments.

Although as a group the RHD speakers produced fewer cues to stress, with correspondingly lower perceptual scores compared to the normal subjects, a great deal of variability is evident within both groups, especially for the normal speakers. The statistical reliability of group differences was tested for each acoustic parameter. The patients were found to produce initial syllables with greater amplitude compared to normal productions, and patients' productions were found to be significantly higher in F_O. No other group effects were obtained, however, suggesting that the production of phonemic stress does not differ significantly between groups. Differences that have been noted, then, are more quantitative in nature than qualitative. That is, although the number of stress cues produced by the RHD patients and the perceptual saliency of stress placement were lower compared to normal subjects' scores, the overall acoustic manifiestations of stress as a function of both syllable position and phrase type did not differ by group.

GENERAL DISCUSSION

The present data corroborate the results of Emmorey (1987), indicating a preserved ability in RHD patients to produce stress contrasts signifying semantic distinctions. Both studies thus contradict the findings of Weintraub and colleagues (1981), who claimed that acoustic cues were absent in the speech of this patient population. The discrepancy in these conclusions may well be due to methodological differences, in that acoustic analyses are more accurate in isolating the prosodic cues from the speech signal. The perceptual scores associated with the tokens produced by RHD patients in the present study may explain the conclusions of Weintraub and colleagues, for stress production was found to be overall less salient compared to normal speakers' productions. Nevertheless, identification scores were above chance, at 66%. Moreover, the manner in which the acoustic correlates to stress patterned as a function of syllable position and phrase type did not differ significantly by group. The present results, then, do not indicate an absence of prosodic cues in the productions of RHD patients.

The results of both Emmorey and the present research may be viewed in light of additional acoustic data (Behrens, 1986) indicating preserved ability in RHD patients to produce sentential emphasis. The same group of patients, reported in the present work as producing phonemic stress, were also found to use the stress cues to signal contrastive stress at the sentence level. Further, perceptual testing showed the placement of sentential emphasis to be more salient, at 77% correct identification, than was production of phonemic stress. Theories of a general dysprosody in RHD populations are thus weakened by the present evidence.

Several problems arise in attempting to verify a theory of general prosodic disorder. At the linguistic level, prosody serves various functions (e.g., semantic distinctions, sentential focus, syntactic structure), and is composed of several acoustic parameters. All these factors must be considered before claiming linguistic deficits. At the emotive level, especially with brain damaged speakers, acoustic analyses are commonly not conducted (although cf. Lieberman & Michaels, 1962; Williams & Stevens, 1972; and Ladd et al., 1985 for data on normal productions of affect); the majority of clinical studies judge emotional quality largely on the basis of the researcher's own impressions of spontaneous and read or imitative speech (e.g., Ross & Mesulam, 1979; Ross, 1981). Further, comprehension abilities are determined through use of intoned stimuli read by the researchers themselves or by hired actors (e.g., Heilman et al., 1975; Ross, 1981). Such artificial situations may fail to tap existing abilities to process affect. It may be that more detailed analysis of both linguistic and emotional stimuli will help to determine the extent to which independent mechanisms exist for propositional and non-propositional prosody.

At present, the results discussed in this chapter suggest a preservation of linguistic prosody in RHD speakers. Viewed in light of emotional dysprosody observed in patients with unilateral right-hemisphere injury, one may infer a dissociation between the control of acoustic parameters to convey linguistic distinctions and to express affect. These results also add support to a growing body of data, from normal subjects (e.g., Behrens, 1985), aphasic patients (e.g., Baum et al., 1982), as well as other investigations with RHD speakers (e.g., Gandour & Dardarananda, 1983), suggesting that the left hemisphere may be superior in the processing of linguistically meaningful prosodic stimuli. An alternative to this linguistic–nonlinguistic distinction for asymmetrical representation, however, is one focused on the domain (local versus global) of prosody. While word stress, a local domain, appears preserved in RHD patients, the integrity of sentence intonation, at the more global level, is less clear for this patient population (e.g., Cooper, et al., 1984; Shapiro & Danly, 1985; Behrens, 1986). Future work needs to consider prosody at its many levels and in its various functions.

REFERENCES

Baum, S.R., Daniloff, R., Daniloff, J., & Lewis, J. (1982). Sentence comprehension by Broca's aphasics: Effects of some suprasegmental variables. *Brain and Language,* 17, 261–271.

Behrens, S.J. (1985). The perception of stress and lateralization of prosody. *Brain and Language,* 26, 332–348.

Behrens, S.J. (1986). The role of the right hemisphere in the production of linguistic prosody: An acoustic analysis. *Ph.D. Thesis, Brown University.*

Behrens, S.J. (in press). The role of the right hemisphere in the production of linguistic stress. *Brain and Language.*

Blumstein, S.E., & Goodglass, H. (1972). The perception of stress as a semantic cue in aphasia. *Journal of Speech and Hearing Research,* 15, 800–806.

Bolinger, D.L., & Gerstman, L.J. (1957). Disjuncture as a cue to constructs. *Journal of the Acoustical Society of America,* 29, 778.

Cooper, W.E., Soares, C., Nicol, J., Michelow, D., & Goloskie, S. (1984). Clausal intonation after unilateral brain damage. *Language and Speech,* 27, 17–24.

Emmorey, K.D. (1987). The neurological substrates for prosodic aspects of speech. *Brain and Language,* 30, 305–320.

Fry, D.B. (1955). Duration and intensity as physical correlates of linguistic stress. *Journal of the Acoustical Society of America,* 27, 765–769.

Gandour, J., & Dardarananda, R. (1983). Identification of tonal contrasts in Thai aphasic patients. *Brain and Language,* 18, 98–114.

Heilman, K.M., Scholes, R., & Watson, R.T. (1975). Auditory affective agnosia: Disturbed comprehension of affective speech. *Journal of Neurology, Neurosurgery, and Psychiatry,* 38, 69–72.

Klatt, D. (1976). Linguistic uses of segmental duration in English: acoustic and perceptual evidence. *Journal of the Acoustical Society of America,* 59, 1208–1221.

Ladd, D.R., Silverman, K.E.A., Tolkmitt, F., Bergmann, G., Scherer, K.R. (1985). Evidence for the independent function of intonation contour type, voice quality, and fundamental frequency range in signalling speaker affect. *Journal of the Acoustical Society of America,* 78, 435–444.

Lieberman, P. (1960). Some acoustic correlates of word stress in American English. *Journal of the Acoustic Society of America,* 32, 451–454.

Lieberman, P., Katz, W., Jongman, A., Zimmerman, R., & Miller, M. (1985). Measures of sentence intonation of read and spontaneous speech in American English. *Journal of the Acoustical Society of America, 77*, 649–657.

Lieberman, P., & Michaels, S.B. (1962). Some aspects of fundamental frequency, envelope amplitude and the emotional content of speech. *Journal of the Acoustical Society of America, 34*, 922–927.

McClean, M.D., & Tiffany, W.R. (1973). The acoustic parameters of stress in relation to syllable position, speech loudness, and rate. *Language and Speech, 16*, 283–290.

Monrad-Krohn, G.H. (1947). Dysprosody or altered 'melody of language'. *Brain, 70*, 405–415.

Monrad-Krohn, G.H. (1963). The third element of speech: Prosody and its disorders. In L. Halpern (Ed.), *Problems of Dynamic Neurology*. Jerusalem: Jerusalem Post Press. 101–118.

Oller, D.K. (1973). The effect of position in utterance on speech segment duration in English. *Journal of the Acoustical Society of America, 54*, 1235–1247.

Ross, E.D. (1981). The aprosodias: Functional-anatomical organization of the affective components of language in the right hemisphere. *Archives of Neurology, 38*, 561–569.

Ross, E.D., & Mesulam, M.M. (1979). Dominant language functions of the right hemisphere? Prosody and emotional gesturing. *Archives of Neurology, 36*, 144–148.

Shapiro, B.E., & Danly, M. (1985). The role of the right hemisphere in the control of speech prosody in propositional and affective contexts. *Brain and Language, 25*, 19–36.

Umeda, N. (1982). 'Fundamental frequency decline' is situation dependent. *Journal of Phonetics, 10*, 279–290.

Weintraub, S., Mesulam, M.M., & Kramer, L. (1981). Disturbances in prosody—A right hemisphere contribution to language. *Archives of Neurology, 38*, 742–744.

Williams, C.E., & Stevens, K.N. (1972). Emotions and speech: Some acoustic correlates. *Journal of the Acoustical Society of America, 52*, 1238–1250.

Ultrasound Measurements of Tongue Dorsum Movements in Articulatory Speech Impairments

Eric Keller

I n many cases, cerebral lesions have direct effects upon the motor aspects of speech. In the case of lesions affecting cortical or subcortical areas with prerolandic focus, disturbances characteristic of motoric types of aphasia are typically observed (especially Broca's asphasia), while in the case of lesions affecting the primary motor cortex, the thalamus and the basal ganglia, the pyramidal and extrapyramidal pathways, the cranial nerves and the cerebellum, disturbances typical of various types of dysarthria can be found.

Utterances of motoric types of aphasia are generally characterized by slowness, intermittent phonetic errors, the presence of a large number of substitutions, omissions and additions of phonemes and, less frequently, the incidence of grammatical and lexical disturbances. On the other hand, dysarthric utterances are identified by the continuous presence of phonetic distortions and by the general absence of grammatical or lexical disturbances.

Research on aphasia has traditionally remained in advance of research in dysarthria, essentially because the errors produced by aphasic patients are relatively easy to transcribe and analyze, while the articulatory disturbances of dysarthric subjects are difficult to describe and almost impossible to transcribe. In spite of important attempts to establish perceptual criteria for the various forms of dysarthria (e.g., cerebellar, parkinsonian, or spastic dysarthria: Darley, Aronson, & Brown, 1969, 1975), the contemporary clinician generally cannot distinguish them with certainty. Judged according to Darley and colleagues' criteria, most dysarthric patients present similar perceptual signs, in particular imprecise consonants,

93

monopitch, reduced syllable stress, and hypernasality (cf. tables presented in Darley et al., 1969, 1975).

The instrumental measurement of articulatory movements (i.e., speech kinematics), promises to provide improved tools for the analysis and the diagnosis of speech motor disturbances, including different forms of dysarthria. In combination with the concepts of contemporary motor theory (in particular, action theory; see, e.g., Keller, 1987a, in press a), the main objective of this approach is to identify the control and impairment variables within the speech motor system.

The following discussion focuses on the instrumental and conceptual approach that the author is developing in this context. The ultrasound recording method for tongue dorsum movements in use in the laboratory is summarized, and some measurement parameters for the evaluation of speech motor disturbances are proposed.

METHOD

Instrumentation

The author's approach involves a computerized system for ultrasound measurements of tongue dorsum movements, developed specifically for two speech-control laboratories located in Montreal (Keller & Ostry, 1983). Transducer placement and the recording system are schematized in Figures 6-1, 6-2, and 6-3.

In order to measure tongue dorsum movements, an ultrasound transducer is placed in a vertical position beneath the chin along the inferior midline of the mandible, and the delay is repeatedly measured between the emission of a short ultrasonic burst (4 μs, 3.5 MHz) and the reception of its echo. In the median plane, the transducer is initially placed at a 90° angle to the Frankfort line (a line connecting the inferior margin of the left ocular orbit with the superior margin of the left external auditory meatus). The final adjustment in this plane requires that there be a greater lingual displacement for [ko] as compared to [ku], and for [ka] as compared to [ko] (Keller & Ostry, 1983, p. 310).

At each millisecond interval, a measurement corresponding to the distance between the transducer and the tongue dorsum is obtained. Specifically, a major echo formed at the interface between the linguo-muscular tissue and the ambient air is located within the ultrasound reflections, and the time between burst emission and the reception of this echo is measured. Measurements of this delay, corresponding to the distance between the transducer and the tongue dorsum, as well as the accompanying digitized acoustic signal, are continuously stored in a microcomputer over a period of 4.5 s (adjustable to 12 s).

Once the recording is completed, the kinematic signal is subjected to curve smoothing by means of spline functions. These cubic functions not only permit following the central tendency of the movement, but also

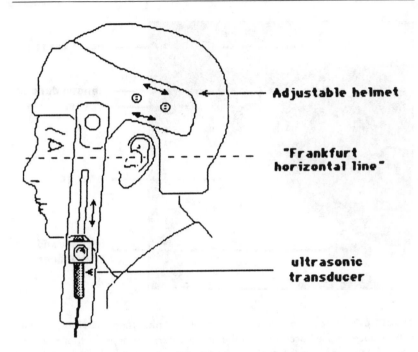

FIGURE 6-1. Ultrasound transducer placement. The transducer is initially placed in vertical position (90° to the Frankfurt horizontal line) at the midline below the inferior mandible, and is adjusted so as to measure successively greater descending movement amplitudes for [ku], [ko], and [ka]. Recordings employing such a helmet attachment have been found to show negligible variability induced by head and mandible movements. (Adapted from Keller & Ostry, 1983.)

provide the first and second derivatives of the tongue displacement; that is, its instantaneous velocity and acceleration (not shown here).

Measurement Variables

On the basis of graphic displays of the ultrasound and voice recordings, several demarkations of the lingual and laryngeal movements are identified in syllables of the type [k + vowel] (see Figure 6-4)[1]. For example, the lingual movement of the syllable [ka] is considered to begin at the point of its highest position prior to movement descent (velocity 0, point 1 on Figure 6-4), the descending movement reaches its maximum velocity at point 2 and terminates at point 4. At point 3, the onset of the

---

[1]For reasons of ultrasound reflection and recording precision, the syllable [ka] provides the most reliable kinematic information using this technology. The recording of more anterior consonants is inhibited by the presence of the anterior sublingual air pocket, and the relatively long lingual movement from [k] to [a] provides a better signal-to-noise ratio than other [k + vowel] combinations, which involve shorter movements.

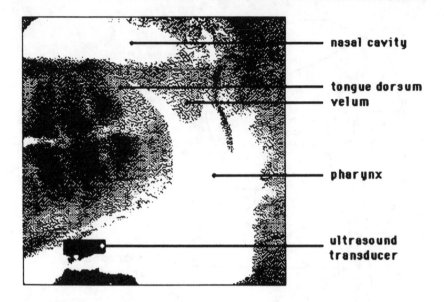

nasal cavity

tongue dorsum
velum

pharynx

ultrasound
transducer

FIGURE 6-2. X-ray of posterior oral, nasal, and pharyngeal cavities, showing a transducer placed according to the noted criteria. It appears that the ultrasound beam traverses the posterior lingual mass in vertical direction and forms an echo at the tissue-air or tissue-saliva interface lying opposite the posterior end of the hard palate.

acoustic effects of the regular vocal cord vibration for vowels can be noted. The ascending movement from the vowel [a] to the consonant [k] starts at the point of lowest position (velocity 0, point 4), reaches its maximum velocity at point 5 and finishes at point 6. In all measurements making reference to points on the velocity curve (all points except point 3), the rightmost measurement is chosen if several measurements are similarly close to zero or to maximum velocity. For point 3, the first glottal pulse in the acoustic voice trace is defined as the first regular pulse deviating from the background noise observed during the preceding linguo-palatal closure. From these reference points, simple calculations of displacement and duration of different sections of the movement provide a number of measurements associated with potential speech motor control variables (see Table 6-1).

Kinematic Variables of Speech Impairment

The specific variables associated with speech motor disturbances are still being investigated. However, recent observations on both normal and abnormal speech (e.g., Keller, 1987b) suggest that the variables presented in Table 6-2 may be useful for more detailed instrumental analyses of speech

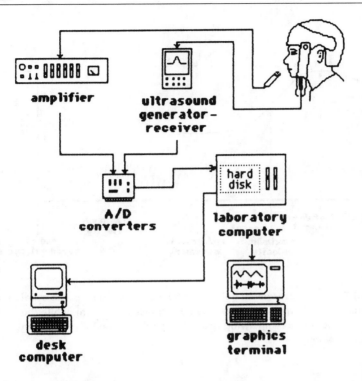

FIGURE 6-3. Present instrumental arrangement. Ultrasound and acoustic data are acquired via an ultrasound generator–receiver and an audio amplifier, are converted to a 1kHz digital signal by a special circuit, and are stored in a laboratory computer. Initial data smoothing and analysis involve the use of a graphics terminal, while statistical evaluations are performed on a disk computer.

motor control. In the next section, cases of disturbances affecting movement extent and regularity, durational extent and regularity, as well as maintenance of movement amplitude, intactness of interarticulatory delays and pathological tremor will be presented. Other possible analyses (not illustrated here) concern movement velocity and its regularity, as well as muscular rigidity.

Task Variables

Three task variables are manipulated in the current protocol: (1) linguistic status; (2) rate of presentation (or syllable duration); and (3) degree of motor habituation. In order to vary linguistic status, the protocol distinguishes the syllable [ka] in the context of normal speech from the diadochokinetic (context free) repetition of the syllable [ka]. The rate of presentation, or syllable duration, is varied, by opposing, in continuous speech, an accentuated syllable (ma*ca*que) to a nonaccentuated syllable

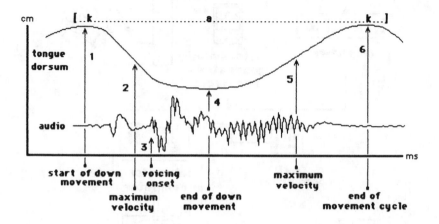

FIGURE 6-4. Measurement points in a typical observation of the syllable [ka]. The top trace shows the tongue dorsum displacement in cm, while the bottom trace shows the accompanying acoustic signal. See text for definitions of the 6 measurement points.

TABLE 6-1. Some Pertinent Measurement Variables

Variable	Definition
Displacement, descending movement	distance 1 - distance 4*
Displacement, ascending movement	distance 4 - distance 6
Displacement to peak velocity, descending	distance 1 - distance 2
Displacement to peak velocity, ascending	distance 4 - distance 5
Cycle duration	time 1 - time 6[†]
Duration, descending movement	time 1 - time 4
Time to peak velocity, descending	time 1 - time 2
Time to peak velocity, ascending	time 4 - time 5
Linguo-laryngeal delay (LLD)	time 1 - time 3
Maximumn velocity, descending movement	velocity at time 2
Maximum velocity, ascending movement	velocity at time 5

*Displacements: a difference of distance *x*—distance *y* refers to the vertical distance in cm traversed by the tongue between point *x* and point *y* in Figure 6-4; e.g., distance 1 – distance 4 corresponds to the vertical displacement between points 1 and 4.

[†]Durations: a difference of time *x* – time *y* refers to the time in ms elapsed between point *x* and point *y* in Figure 6-4; e.g., time 1 – time 6 corresponds to the duration between points 1 and 6.

TABLE 6-2. Some Impairment Variables

Impairment Variable	Estimator
Movement amplitude	Mean of displacement, descending movement
Movement duration	Mean of duration, descending movement
Variability of movement amplitude	Coefficient of variation* of displacement, descending movement
Variability of movement duration	Coefficient of variation* of duration, descending movement
Variability of cycle duration	Coefficient of variation* of cycle duration
Variability of interarticulatory coordination	Coefficient of variation* of linguo-laryngeal delay (LLD)
Maintenance of movement amplitude	Degree of decrease in successive displacements, descending movement
Movement velocity	Mean of maximum velocity, descending movement
Differentiation of long and short movement amplitudes	Ratio of displacements for long and short descending movements
Differentiation of long and short movement durations	Ratio of durations for long and short descending movements
Rigidity	Slope of the linear relation between the displacement of the descending movement and its maximum velocity
Tremor	An important presence of information in the movement spectrum between 6 and 12 Hz.

*Coefficient of variation = SD/mean.

(lac à canards)[2], and in the diadochokinetic repetition, by contrasting normal and fast utterance rates (see Table 6-3). Finally, the degree of motor habituation is varied by asking the subject to produce the stimulus protocol twice; once normally and once with clenched teeth.

Between 20 and 40 samples of the syllable [ka] for each of the eight conditions are obtained by means of this protocol. A recording session takes about 45 minutes, including ultrasound transducer adjustments, stimulus presentation, and recording.

---

[2]No French context could be found in which the syllable [ka], embedded between two other [ka]-syllables, does not cross a morpheme boundary. However, once a smooth delivery is established, no phonetic effect of the morpheme boundary could be discerned in the speech of subjects and patients recorded to date.

TABLE 6-3. Task Variables

	Contextfree Repetition	Repetition in Linguistic Context
Normal speech rate/ long vowel(s)	. . . ka*ka*ka . . . [. . ka:*ka*:ka: . . .]	le ma*ca*que assommé [. . ka:*ka*:ka: . . .]
Fast speech rate/short vowels(s)	. . . ka*ka*ka . . . [. . ka*ka*ka . . .]	le la*c à* canards [. . ka*ka*ka . . .]

ARTICULATORY SPEECH IMPAIRMENTS

The Reference Norm: A Randomly Selected Normal Subject

To illustrate the recordings of a normal case, data from a subject chosen randomly among the 12 normal subjects recently recorded in our laboratory are presented here: a 23-year-old francophone, female, of middle-class background, and free of known linguistic disturbances. Figure 6-5a shows vertical lingual movements for the repetition of context-free [ka], produced at a subject-paced, normal utterance rate.

Several aspects can be noted in Figure 6-5. First, the extent and duration of the descending movements are quite regular. Also, descending movements are rapid and always carried out without hesitation, while the ascending movement is often executed with a hesitation occurring between the lowest point and the final part of the ascension towards the highest point of the movement (points C on Figure 6-5a). A comparison of this illustration with the next figure (Figure 6-5b) indicates that the presence of such *platforms* is one of a number of variables (such as extent and duration of movement) that distinguishes slower from more rapid productions of [ka] in the speech of this subject.

Further, it can be seen that the coordination between lingual movement and laryngal activity is rather regular in the normal subject. The onset of laryngal activity (the B points on Figure 6-5a) follows the beginning of the lingual activity (the A points) within a predictable delay (40–60 ms in fast-rate conditions and 80–150 ms in normally paced conditions).

Finally, it is possible to observe a preparatory movement prior to the articulation of the stimulus syllables (point D). This movement regularly preceeds the descending movement associated with the first syllable [ka]. Its likely function is to provide the subsequent descending movement with sufficient momentum to produce a satisfactory air plosion in opening from [k] to [a].

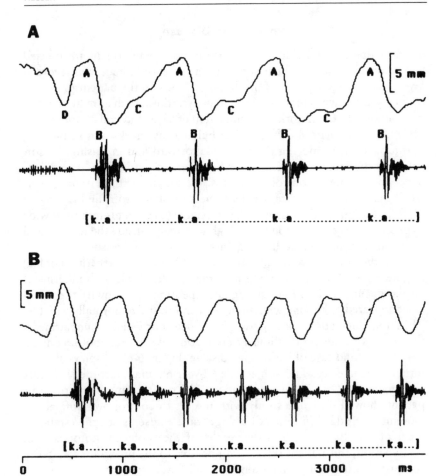

FIGURE 6-5. Tongue dorsum movements and acoustic wave forms in context-free repetitions of [ka] by a randomly selected normal subject. A = point of linguo-palatal contact; B = onset of regular glottal pulse oscillation visible in the audio track; C = "hesitation platform" during ascending movement (corresponding to syllable offset); D = preparatory movement prior to first articulated syllable.

Movements associated with a fast production of [ka] (e.g., Figure 6-5b) differ from those of slow movements primarily with respect to duration. The short syllables produced by this subject lasted about 500 ms, while the long syllables measured approximately 900 ms. In context-free speech production, this time reduction tends to be associated primarily with a modification of the ascending movement.

Parkinson's Disease

The first two individuals with speech-motor impairment are affected by Parkinson's disease. The first patient, a 63-year-old man, was recorded 5 years after the diagnosis of his illness. To the ear, the patient presented certain well-known signs of parkinsonian dysarthria, such as reduced stress and monopitch. On Dworkin's examination of facial and oral motor control (1978), he experienced difficulties in bulging his cheeks and in blowing into a balloon, in moving the mandible forward and in raising the soft palate for the production of [a]. Yet the same examination showed no disturbance in the motor control of the lips, the tongue or the larynx. Let us recall that in the lingual tasks, the subject must (1) protrude his tongue; (2) follow a tongue-depressor with his tongue; (3) open his mouth as wide as possible and raise his tongue as high as possible inside the mouth; and (4) push with his tongue hard against the tongue depressor.

On the other hand, the ultrasound recording of slow repetition of [ka] (Figure 6-6A) shows an irregular movement, measurable both in terms of displacement and duration. During fast repetition (not shown), the movement appeared to be somewhat more regular, but still abnormally variable. Thus, the kinematic recording was able to detect articulatory impairments that were not evident in a clinical examination of orofacial motor control.

The second case of Parkinson's disease (Figure 6-6b) displays another form of disturbance. This subject is a 62-year-old man, recorded six years post-diagnosis. On clinical examination of his orofacial motor control, this patient showed difficulties only with respect to control over soft palate movements. Judged in terms of his age, time elapsed since the establishment of the diagnosis, and the results of the orofacial motor control examination, this patient seemed comparable to the previous case. Yet in contrast, his ultrasound recording showed few irregularities.

On the other hand, he presented a pronounced lack of coordination between lingual and laryngeal activity; Figure 6-6b shows that the vocal cords were frequently vibrating at the very moment that the tongue touched the palate for the consonant [k] (confirmed by zoom-type verifications of detailed segments of the articulation, not shown here). All the same, the auditory impression of the consonant articulations of this recording remained consistent with the stop [k]. This disturbance is likely to be of clinical relevance because this type of dyscoordination has never been observed in any of our normal francophone or anglophone subjects.

Senile Dementia

The following observations concern a 68-year-old woman with senile dementia. Among the visible signs of her motor disturbance, there was a severe tremor of the inferior mandible, both during speech production

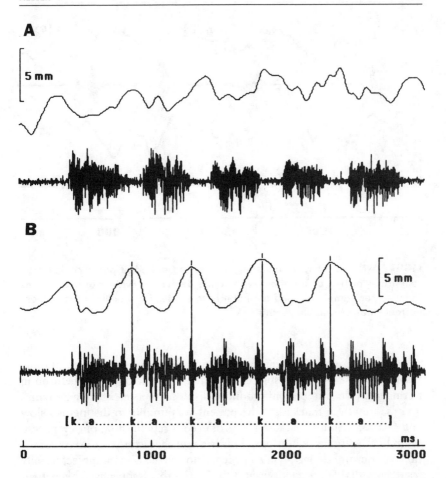

FIGURE 6-6. (A) Normally-paced contextfree repetition of [ka] by a patient with Parkinson's disease. Articulations were highly irregular, even though the orofacial motor control examination showed no disturbance of tongue movements. (B) Fast contextfree repetition of [ka] in another patient with Parkinson's disease. In 3 out of 4 articulations, the point of linguo-palatal closure coincided with vocal cord activity, yet the auditory impression remained consistent with a dysarthric production of the stop [k].

and at rest. Furthermore, this person talked with a harsh, low voice, and with distorted articulation. She also persevered beyond the 4.5-second recording periods by repeating stimulus sequences such as *le macaque assommé* or *le lac à canards* for up to several minutes subsequent to the recording. In addition, she walked slowly and with difficulty.

The ultrasound recording analysis (Figures 6-7a and 6-7b) shows a severe lingual motor control disturbance. First, there is a general irregularity

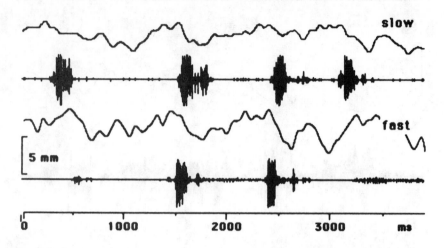

FIGURE 6-7. Normally paced (*slow*) and (supposedly) fast-paced context-free repetitions of [ka] by a patient with senile dementia. Evident are reductions in movement amplitude and an inability to produce distinctively faster-than-normal rates of syllable repetition.

of movement, with a substantial reduction in the movement's amplitude. Instead of an 8–10 mm displacement, characteristic of slow repetition in normal subjects, this patient produced displacements measuring 2–3 mm, and maximally 6 mm. Also, the patient was unable to distinguish slow and fast repetition rates, and she produced a repetition about every 900 ms in both stimulus conditions. This is a rate characteristic of slow repetition in a normal subject, while fast repetition in the normal subject usually results in syllable productions at 3 to 5 times this frequency. This patient thus appears to have selective difficulties in programming the motor parameters of fast speech production.

Finally, a spectral analysis of several of her lingual movements was performed, in order to verify if tongue movements were also affected by tremor. In normal subjects, voluntary repetitions of the syllable [ka] usually occur at a 0.5 to 6 Hz rhythm, while involuntary, tremorlike movements are usually reported to be substantially faster (6 to 12 Hz). A spectral analysis (Fast Fourier Transform) can distinguish slower and faster regular movements by showing their frequency in the form of amplitude peaks within a display of the movement's temporal components.

The results of this analysis were somewhat ambiguous (see Figure 6-8). Although certain peaks were visible between 8 and 10 Hz, their amplitude was inferior to the one usually associated with tremor (see, e.g., Hunker & Abbs, 1984). Thus, it was concluded that the involuntary movement elements noted in this spectral analysis were most probably secondary

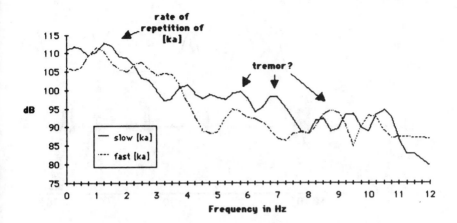

FIGURE 6-8. A spectral analysis of two typical 2048-ms segments of tongue dorsum movement for contextfree, normally paced (*slow*) and fast repetitions of [ka] by the patient with senile dementia (cf. Fig. 6-7). The peaks at 1.1 and 1.2 Hz correspond to the patient's rate of syllable repetition in the two utterance segments, while peaks at around 6, 7, and 9 Hz correspond to involuntary, regular movement superimposed on the articulatory movements.

consequences of the severe inferior jaw tremor, and were not representative of lingual tremor *per se*. In view of the prominent hypothesis that suggests a central origin of the oscillatory motor commands for tremor (e.g., Hassler, Mundinger, & Riechert, 1970), it is possible that at such a central level, the jaw musculature is controlled independently of the lingual musculature.

Adult Stuttering

The next case concerns the motor effects of stuttering. Several explorations of the speech impairments of stutterers have been performed in our laboratory. For instance, in comparing two adolescent severe stutterers to normal controls, Garcia (1981) observed that displacements of the syllable [ka] were significantly more variable in the stutterers than in the normal subjects.

While this irregularity is less obvious in the repetition of the stimulus [k'akə], produced by a 40-year-old anglophone stutterer with mild impairment (Figure 6-9), other distubances can be noted in this subject. First, the initial movement seems exaggerated in comparison with normal subjects' initial movements (see Figures 6-5a and 6-5b). This observation can be related to the common observation that the initial syllable of a stuttered utterance tends to be more impaired than non-initial syllables. Figure 6-9 also shows that the amplitude of lingual movements decreases over

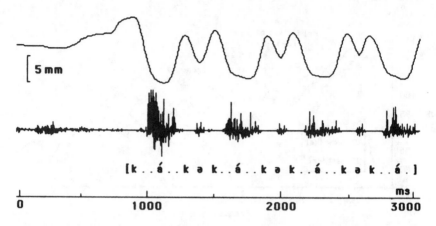

FIGURE 6-9. Tongue movements in a repetition of [k′akə] by an adult anglophone speaker with a mild stuttering impairment. Evident are an excessive movement amplitude (1.3 mm) for the initial syllable, an insufficient distinction of movement amplitudes for stressed [k′a] and unstressed [kə] syllables, and a decrease of kinematic abnormalities with successive articulations.

stimulus repetitions, which is an unknown phenomenon in normal subjects.

Another motor difficulty lies in the distinction between the short movements of the [kə] syllable and the long movements of the [k′a] syllable. While normal anglophone subjects' short movements tend to measure between ⅓ and ¼ of the amplitude of long movements (not illustrated here), the three stuttering subjects recorded in our laboratory produced *short* movements measuring about ⅔ of the amplitude of *long* movements. Figure 6-9 indicates that the difference between the two types of movement becomes more pronounced with each stimulus repetition, again indicating that motor control improves over several postinitial repetitions of the same stimulus.

These findings on excessive variability, decreasing movement amplitude, and insufficient distinction of movement amplitudes for short and long syllables are comparable to observations commonly made with patients affected by neurological lesions. Although it is evident that the generality of stutterers are not affected by gross neurological lesions, these results do support the hypothesis that their articulation difficulties are related to a still ill-defined imbalance of neuromotor control. If at some future point it can be established that these signs are the exclusive consequence of neurological lesions, this type of observation would support the notion of a constitutional origin of stuttering (see e.g., Sussman & MacNeilage, 1975; Wood, Stump, McKeehan, Sheldon, & Proctor, 1980).

Probable Cranial Traumatism

The last case, affected by a particularly mild speech impairment, was referred for instrumental speech evaluation by his neurologist in order to establish if he was indeed suffering from a measurable speech motor control disturbance. He was a 65-year-old retired truck driver who had hit his head 16 years ago in a fall on a delivery platform. At the time of the accident, no mnesic loss was noted, but during the 8 days following the accident, he was, according to self-report, unable to speak. The medical history notes a probable subdural hematoma over the left hemisphere, but at the time no CT-scan was taken. A recently taken CT-scan was normal, suggesting that whatever neuological lesion may have been present at the time of the accident, may in the meanwhile have been resorbed.

His present conversational speech is normal, but when he tires, his voice amplitude fades. Moreover, he complains that "it stutters" when he talks fast. The clinical examination indicated a very slight orofacial motor control problem: for instance, the patient could not touch his superior lip with his tongue, while remaining capable of turning it towards his chin. He also had difficulty in alternating 2 oral movements (kissing and tongue clicking). He had difficulties in maintaining lateral pressure against a tongue depressor to the right; furthermore, he pushed vertically against the tongue depressor with apparently spastic strength.

The instrumental examination revealed impairments that had not been evident to the ear (Figures 6-10A and 6-10B). Irregular movements can be noted, particularly along the temporal axis, as well as progressive decreases in movement amplitude in fast repetition (Figure 6-10B). A statistical evaluation revealed that measures of movement duration were consistently more variable than those of normal controls (Figure 6-11A and 6-11B). This was especially true of syllable duration, which when analyzed by coefficients of variation (SD/mean), was between 2.3 and 2.7 times more variable than those of normal subjects (exception: short, unaccented [ka] in "le lac à canards"). None of the 12 normal francophone and 2 normal anglophone subjects tested with the same protocol showed anywhere near that degree of variability on these durational variables. At the same time, movement amplitudes or velocities were by and large not different from those of control subjects. These results will be reported in greater detail in Keller, Cot, & Labrecque (in preparation).

On the basis of this information, it was concluded that this patient's probable cranial traumatism, suffered 16 years ago, indeed affects his speech motor control to some degree. A selective programming error for the temporal variables of speech motor control is in evidence, which affects the patient's ability to maintain regular syllable rhythm throughout the utterance.

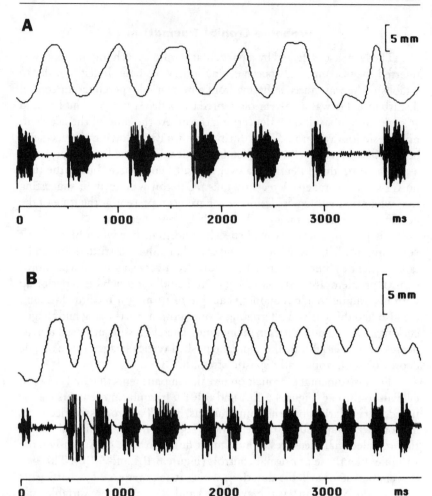

FIGURE 6-10. Normally paced (*slow*) and fast contextfree repetitions of [ka] by a patient (RD) affected by a cranial trauma probably experienced 16 yrs. prior to recording. Although the speech of this patient was essentially normal, ultrasound recordings showed (A) a selective disturbance of durational variables, and (B) a decrease of movement amplitudes over successive articulations.

CONCLUSIONS

These observations permit a number of methodological and clinical conclusions. First, it appears that the ultrasound evaluation of lingual motor control constitutes a promising methodology in the analysis of speech neuromotor disturbances. Several cases presented here showed only minimal

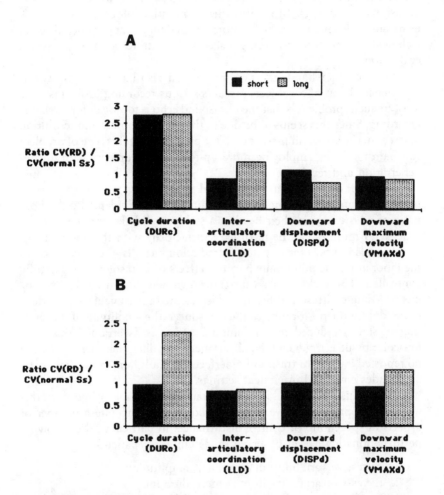

FIGURE 6-11. (cf. Figure 6-10) Patient RD's variability on various measurements, as compared with the average variability shown by normal subjects (A: context-free repetition of [ka], B: [ka] in linguistic context). The statistic used is the ratio of the respective coefficients of variation (s.d./mean); e.g., a ratio of 2.7 on cycle duration shows that patient RD was 2.7 times more variable than the average normal subject with respect to this measurement parameter.

disturbances in the clinical examination for speech and orofacial motor control, while severe speech motor disturbances were clearly evident in the ultrasound recordings. Moreover, the quantitative information available by means of this method is by far more detailed than that obtained through a clinical examination, rendering it accessible to more extensive statistical evaluation.

On the other hand, the present method also has its limits. In our experience, 1 out of 5 subjects presents serious recording problems. The most frequent problem is that the ultrasound echo is too weak for a reliable recording. Since this seems to be due to the limits of power and resolution inherent in the system in present use, it is probable that this type of problem can be resolved by employing more up-to-date instruments with greater penetration and resolution.

Another difficulty has been noted with respect to the tremor, or involuntary movements, present in certain patients. Evidently, only those patients who can hold their head in a stable, well-balanced position for at least 15 minutes can be recorded satisfactorily with this method.

It is also important to consider radiation hazards in this context. In the laboratory, the potentially harmful effects of ultrasound are carefully controlled. The Picker A-scan instrument, model 103, used operates by means a single ultrasound beam and is destined for clinical use. Furthermore, during the positioning of the transducer, the amplitude of the emitting crystal is reduced to a minimum, and it is ascertained that only muscular tissue is irradiated. Finally, is merits recalling that there have been no reported harmful ultrasound bioeffects on adult humans at diagnostic amplitudes employed in clinical settings.

In conclusion, several kinematic parameters available by means of this method can probably serve to assess and further elucidate a number of aspects of speech motor control disturbance. In particular, the following perturbations have been observed in a number of patients:

1. Excessive variability in movement amplitude
2. Excessive variability in movement duration
3. Insufficient coordination between different articulatory organs
4. Insufficient maintenance of movement amplitude throughout an utterance
5. Insufficient spatial and temporal differentiation of short and long movements
6. Perhaps the presence of tremor superimposed upon the lingual movement.

In further research, it will be explored if it is possible to reliably associate these deficits with specific syndromes, and it will be attempted to integrate these observations with current theory of human motor control. It is hoped that this type of measurement of speech articulation will permit rational and theoretically sound associations between observations on speech motor disturbances on the one hand, and findings on normal speech motor control on the other.

ACKNOWLEDGMENTS

The author wishes to thank Anne Simon and Françoise Cot, speech therapists, for performing clincial examinations of orofacial motor control in 3 of the patients presented, as well as Drs. Serge Gauthier, Jean-François Demonet, and Raymonde Labrecque for referring a number of these cases to me for instrumental analysis. Also, thanks to Ginette Ladouceur for performing various data and statistical analyses. Finally, particular thanks are due to Monique Daoust, whose translation of the author's French-language address to the Société Québecoise de recherches en psychologie (Nov. 1985), forms the basis of this text. This research is supported by the National Science and Engineering Council of Canada (NSERC) (Grant A1034), by the F.C.A.R.–Quebec (team 128), by the "Programme de l'aide financière aux chercheurs et aux créateurs" (P.A.F.A.C.C) of the Université du Québec à Montréal and by the Medical Research Council of Canada (M.R.C.C.) (Grant PG-28 to the Centre de Recherche, CHCN).

REFERENCES

Darley, F.L., Aronson, A.E., & Brown, J.R. (1969). Differential diagnostic patterns of dysarthria. *Journal of Speech and Hearing Research, 12,* 246–269.
Darley, F.L., Aronson, A.E., & Brown, J.R. (1975). *Motor speech disorders.* Philadelphia: W.B. Saunders.
Dworkin, J.P. (1978). II. Differential diagnosis of motor speech disorders: The clinical examination of the speech mechanism. *Journal of National Student Speech and Hearing Association, December,* 37–62.
Garcia, L. (1981). *Ultrasonic measurement of tongue displacement in stutterers* (Masters degree project, McGill University).
Hassler, R., Mundinger, F., & Reichert, T. (1970). Pathophysiology of tremor at rest derived from the correlation of anatomical and clinical data. *Confinia Neurologica, 32,* 79–87.
Hunker, C.J., & Abbs, J.H. (1984). Physiological analyses of parkinsonian tremors in the orofacial system. In M.R. McNeil, J.C. Rosenbek, & A.E. Aronson (Eds.), *The dysarthrias: Physiology, acoustics, perception, management.* San Diego, CA: College-Hill Press, pp. 69–100.
Keller, E. (1987a). The cortical representation of motor processes of speech. In E. Keller, & M. Gopnik (Eds.), *Motor and sensory processes of language.* Hillsdale, NJ: Lawrence Erlbaum Associates, pp. 125–162.
Keller, E. (1987b). Factors underlying tongue articulation in speech. *Journal of Speech and Hearing Research, 30,* 223–229.
Keller, E. (in press). Analyse fonctionnelle des perturbations neurologiques de

la mortricité de la parole. In H. Cohen (Ed.), *Perspectives contemporaines en neuroscience*. Montréal: Études Vivantes.

Keller, E., Cot, F., & Labrecque, R. (in preparation). A case of selective impairment of temporal aspects of speech articulation.

Keller, E., & Ostry, D. (1983). Computerized pulsed echo ultrasound measurements of tongue dorsum movements. *Journal of the Acoustical Society of America, 73,* 1309–1315.

Sussman, H.M., & MacNeilage, P.F. (1975). Hemispheric specializaton for speech production and perception in stutterers. *Neuropsychologia, 13,* 19–26.

Wood, F., Stump, D., McKeehan, A., Sheldon, S., & Proctor, J. (1980). Patterns of regional cerebral blood flow during attempted reading aloud by stutteres both on and off haloperidol medication: Evidence for inadequate left frontal activation during stuttering. *Brain and Language, 9,* 141–144.

Electropalatographic Study of Articulation Disorders in Verbal Dyspraxia

W.J. Hardcastle

There is considerable disagreement in the literature as to the precise nature of neurogenic disorders affecting primarily the production of speech, such as verbal dyspraxia (or apraxia of speech) (see reviews in Lesser, 1978; Rosenbek, Kent, & La Pointe, 1984; Edwards, 1984). This classic description of the disorder and one that is widely used by clinicians is that proposed by Darley and his associates (Darley 1967; 1982; Deal & Darley, 1972). In this view the disorder is seen primarily as a motor programming disorder, or more specifically an articulation problem resulting from an impairment in the capacity to program the positioning of the speech musculature for speech sounds and to produce smooth transitions between muscle movements. The speech output that results is described impressionistically as "effortful" and is frequently accompanied by *groping* or *searching* movements of the oral structures. There are inconsistent and variable articulatory errors with apparent substitutions, additions, repetitions, and prolongations of sounds usually in excess of omissions or distortions and these occur most noticeably in spontaneous volitional speech rather than in automatic or reflexive acts, and the degree of disintegration is in direct proportion to the length and complexity of the utterance, multisyllabic words being most vulnerable. Unlike in the dysarthrias, the speech musculature does not show significant weakness, slowness or incoordination when used for reflexive and automatic acts. Attempts at self-correction are frequent and usually successful.

Other investigators claim it is difficult to account for many of the dyspraxic errors solely in terms of articulatory motor programming. Some stress for example that the errors are rule-governed and can be described according to a phonological system (see, e.g., Blumstein, 1973; Martin &

113

Rigrodsky, 1974: Trost & Canter, 1974). Trost and Canter (1974) for example in a study of apraxia of speech in patients with Broca's aphasia noted a number of regular tendencies; for example, vowels were produced more accurately than consonants, single consonants more accurately than clusters, most errors differed from the target by only one or two distinctive features, place distinctions were most affected, and initial position caused most problems.

Another complicating factor in the description of the disorder is that pure forms of verbal dyspraxia are quite rare, the disorder usually being accompanied by some aphasic symptoms. These may include agrammatism, paraphasia and other disturbances in language production and comprehension. One of the problems for the clinician is to identify the dyspraxic element if it exists. If dyspraxia is deemed to be present, appropriate therapy for a motor programming type problem would then be carried out—such as developing articulatory coordination, or placement of speech organs for specific sounds—strategies that would be largely irrelevant for an aphasic type disorder. It is important, therefore, before devising appropriate treatment programs, to understand the nature of the disorder. Such an understanding will only come however from more objective and precise descriptions of the speech characteristics of the disorder itself than are traditionally available. It will not be sufficient, for example, simply to label an error a phoneme "substitution" or "distortion" as is traditionally done. We need to identify precisely the activities of the speech organs and the way in which they interact to produce the manifestly abnormal speech output. In other words we need to assess the underlying reason for the perceived substitution or distortion. Thus a /k/ heard in initial position instead of a /t/ in a word like *tick* may have at least two interpretations. One possibility is that the /k/ phoneme has been wrongly selected at a hypothetical higher-level linguistic encoding stage in the generation of the utterance and has been produced correctly with the appropriate vocal tract configuration for the velar stop. An alternative interpretation is that the appropriate articulatory gestures for the phonemes have been correctly selected, but at a later stage of neural processing the serial ordering of these gestures has become disturbed so that the raising of the body of the tongue appropriate for the /k/ occurs prematurely in relation to the initial tongue tip gesture for the /t/ and a double alveolar–velar stop results, sounding in this case more like a /k/ than a /t/. This could then be seen primarily as a problem in the sequencing of articulatory gestures rather than an incorrect selection of phonemes (a similar case involving the phasing of velum and tongue tip is discussed by Itoh and Sasanuma, 1984). The important point is that a substitution error, /k/ for /t/ is perceived by the listener— and the speaker did not correct it. The auditory-based judgment in this case therefore may not be very illuminating as it reveals nothing of the intricate events that take place during speech production, the complex overlapping movements of the articulators (e.g., coarticulation), and the transitional movements between target vocal configurations, although it is precisely these details of the dynamics of speech organs that may be crucial diagnostically. In fact, the use of discrete symbols in an auditory-based transcription may give a quite misleading impression as by its very nature it often forces the listener into making categorical decisions about speech sounds, e.g., whether an articulatory event is to be represented as a /t/ or a /k/.

Quite apart from its inadequacy in representing as it does only the peripheral output of the speech production process, the auditory-based analysis will be limited in other ways. It is inherently unreliable, dependent as it is on many uncontrollable factors such as the transcriber's own skill, type of training, etc. Even under optimum listening conditions with multiple playback facilities it has been shown that skilled transcribers can only expect about 70% level of agreement in the choice of symbols in the representation of disordered speech (see Amorosa et al., 1985).

In recent years investigators have begun to turn from sole reliance on impressionistic descriptions to relatively more objective methods of analysis using instrumental techniques for investigating acoustic, aerodynamic and physiological aspects of verbal dyspraxia (see, e.g., review in Rosenbek et al., 1984). Kent and Rosenbek (1983), for example, identified a number of measurable acoustic characteristics of verbal dyspraxia including slow-speaking rate with lengthening of both transitional and steady states of the acoustic signal, relative flattening of prosodic constrasts, slow and inaccurate movements of articulators, initiation difficulties, discoordination of voicing with other articulators. Duffy and Gawle (1984) measured vowel duration preceding voiced and voiceless consonants and found apraxics in general differentiated the duration in the same way as normals but with some overlap in values and considerable variability. The abnormal distribution of values was interpreted by the authors as being a consequence of generally shortened vowels in a context of poor precision of temporal control, but that accurate phonological selection of the voicing feature is intact (Duffy & Gawle, 1984). Evidence for this temporal variability has come also from studies of the Voice Onset Time (VOT) distinctions used by dyspraxic speakers (see, e.g., Blumstein et al, 1980; Itoh & Sasanuma, 1984). Physiological studies, e.g., the X-ray microbeam study of Itoh and Sasanuma (1984), have found evidence of discoordination of timing among several articulators such as the velum, lip, and tongue. The authors conclude that dyspraxia is associated with a breakdown of the normally tight temporal patterning of the component movements in a transition. Such temporal discoordination can lead to perceptual distortion. These studies have provided valuable data but most are limited by the nature of the instrumentation and the relatively small number of subjects. There is obviously a pressing need for further objective studies using a wide range of instrumental techniques to identify the speech characteristics of dyspraxia and to differentiate it from other disorders that have some features in common with it such as aphasia and dysarthria.

A technique that has considerable potential for offering new insights into the nature of errors in dyspraxic speech is Electropalatography (EPG). This technique records spatial and temporal details of tongue contact with the hard palate during continuous speech, thus providing qualitative and quantitative data on a feature that has considerable phonetic relevance, namely the place of articulation. In the present system, the subject wears a thin acrylic plate, .8 mm thick, moulded to fit tightly against the hard palate and containing 62 silver electrodes mounted on the surface (for details see Hardcastle, 1984; Hardcastle et al, 1985). When contact occurs between the tongue and any of these electrodes a signal is conducted via lead-out wires to an external processing unit that enables the patterns of contact to be stored in a microprocessor and displayed on a video monitor screen. Permanent records of the contact patterns can be obtained from a computer print-out for further, more detailed, analysis.

An examination of EPG data for a variety of speech sounds produced by normal speakers has indicated that most lingual consonants including /t, d, n, s, z, ʃ, ʒ, k, g, ŋ, tʃ, dʒ/ and front close or half-close vocalic elements such as /i, ɛ, eɪ, aɪ/ show measurable amounts of lingual-palatal contact during some stage of their production. EPG is ideally suited for measuring the dynamic patterns of such contacts, e.g., the changes in contact patterns during the approach and release phases of obstruents as well as target configurations during the constriction phase. Also, although the technique does not indicate precisely which part of the tongue touches the palate, reasonable inferences can be made from a study of the contact patterns themselves in relation to the actual shape of the individual palate, and a general background knowledge of the anatomy and physiology of the tongue gained from dissection work (e.g., Miyawaki, 1974) and the results of X-ray and electromyographic investigations (e.g., Alfonso & Baer, 1982).

In the present study, the system is used to record details of tongue contact during production of a variety of isolated words by a speaker described as verbal dyspraxic. All the items are transcribed with a narrow phonetic transcription system and the patterns of contact compared with a normal speaker's.

METHOD

Subject

BT is a male, aged 49, who suffered a left hemisphere CVA in November 1983 leaving him initially mute, a condition that resolved over the following weeks into a moderate Broca's type aphasia. The Boston

Diagnostic Aphasia Examination was carried out in December 1983, February and September 1984, and the latest results are given as follows: Melodic line 6–7; phrase length 7 words; articulatory agility, 5; grammatical form 7: paraphasia 7 (absent); word finding 4 (information proportional to fluency); comprehension 7 (normal). His speech at the time of the present study was therefore diagnosed as that of a mild dyspraxia, characterized impressionistically by nonfluency with disturbed prosody and "sound searching." Automatic speech was functional and fluent and his general severity (4 on the Boston scale) was that of loss of fluency in speech without significant limitation of ideas expressed or their form of expression. His auditory comprehension was assessed to be within normal limits (Four adult native speakers of English served as controls, providing EPG data which were compared with BT's patterns).

Corpus

The test material consisted of 50 single word items. These are arranged in three lists (see Appendix 7-1). Lists A and B contain the lingual consonants of English in a variety of phonetic environments and in word initial and final positions. List C contains sequences of consonants of varying degrees of complexity both within a single morpheme and across morpheme boundaries. All items were presented to the subjects as flash cards that contain both the word written in orthography and a pictorial representation. The subjects were instructed to preface each word with the indefinite article which was manifested phonetically either as [ə] or [eɪ]. Each subject produced at least four repetitions of the word list over a period of several weeks with the experimenter taking care to ensure the recording conditions were as similar as practicable on successive occasions.

Procedure

Each subject was fitted with an artificial palate for the EPG study. The electrodes were arranged according to a predetermined scheme of placement based on anatomical landmarks (see Hardcastle et al., 1987) to enable comparisons in contact patterns to be made between subjects. Prior to the recording sessions subjects wore a dummy plate without the electrodes but of the same thickness as the real plate for increasing periods of time, including at least one 24-hour period, so as to become accustomed to the feel of the device in the mouth.

Permanent records of the tongue–palate contacts were obtained in the form of computer print-outs for the four repetitions of each word by all subjects. Analyses were based on these print-outs.

Figure 7-1 shows an artificial palate used for EPG, a print-out of contact patterns that occur during a normal subject's production of the

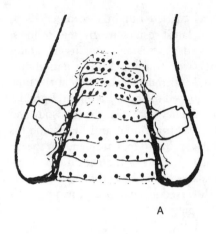

A

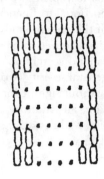

B

C

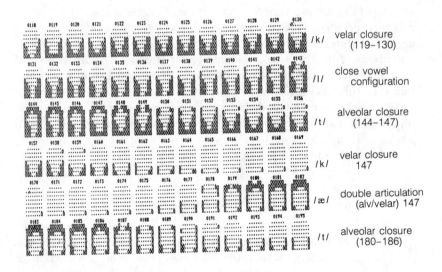

| | | | | | | | | | | | | | | |
|0118|0119|0120|0121|0122|0123|0124|0125|0126|0127|0128|0129|0130| /k/ | velar closure (119–130) |

| 0131|0132|0133|0134|0135|0136|0137|0138|0139|0140|0141|0142|0143| /l/ | close vowel configuration |

| 0144|0145|0146|0147|0148|0149|0150|0151|0152|0153|0154|0155|0156| /t/ | alveolar closure (144–147) |

| 0157|0158|0159|0160|0161|0162|0163|0164|0165|0166|0167|0168|0169| /k/ | velar closure 147 |

| 0170|0171|0172|0173|0174|0175|0176|0177|0178|0179|0180|0181|0182| /æ/ | double articulation (alv/velar) 147 |

| 0183|0184|0185|0186|0187|0188|0189|0190|0191|0192|0193|0194|0195| /t/ | alveolar closure (180–186) |

FIGURE 7-1. An artificial palate used for EPG (A) and a computer print-out of lingual–palatal contacts during production of the word *kitkat* [kʰɪtkæt] (C). Sample interval is 10 ms and frames are numbered from left to right. In each palate diagram the electrode positions are arranged schematically as in the single frame (B).

118

word *kitkat* and a schematic representation of a single palatal frame (A). The schematic representation shows the palate divided up into convenient reference zones based on phonetic place categories. In (B) electrode rows 1–3 (from the top) represent the alveolar zone; rows 4–5, the palatal zone; and rows 6–8, the velar zone. In the print-out for *kitkat* (C) each palate diagram is 10 ms apart and the sequence of tongue contacts during the word (represented by zeros) is read from left to right.

RESULTS OF EPG INVESTIGATION

Single Consonant Data

ALVEOLAR STOPS AND NASALS. Most of BT's deviations from normal patterns involved the oral stop targets in word initial position. The patterns produced by BT were very inconsistent with velar closure (i.e., complete contact across the posterior row of electrodes) sometimes accompanying the anterior alveolar contact. Figures 7-2, 7-3, and 7-4 illustrate this double articulation pattern with computer print-outs of tongue-palate contacts for the initial stops in the three words *tickling* (2nd rep.), *deer* (4th rep.), and *dart* (4th rep.). The other repetitions of these words did not show the velar contact pattern. In each case the normal pattern is reproduced above BT's for comparison. The initial stop in *tickling* was transcribed as a prolonged [t], but those in *deer* and *dart* were heard as [gd]. In *tickling* the double velar–alveolar pattern occurs after the onset of the alveolar stop, but in *deer* and *dart* the velar closure precedes the alveolar closure. This double-closure pattern never occurred for the normal speakers in this context. On two repetitions of *dolls* BT produced a velar stop without any anterior closure which was then corrected to a normal /d/ pattern (see Figure 7-5). Apart from these abnormalities the alveolar stops and all nasals were perceived as normal and produced with normal anterior closure patterns although in general with prolonged duration of the closure phase.

VELAR STOP AND NASAL. Most velar stops and nasals were produced normally in initial and final positions except for two repetitions of *leg* where alveolar closure (heard as [d]) occurred instead of the target velar. On one occasion this error was corrected to the required velar stop pattern for the /g/. In general BT's stops had a longer closure phase than the normals.

LATERAL APPROXIMANT. BT produced normal patterns for all /l/ targets with anterior closure and evidence of bilateral release. The auditory impression was a normal [l].

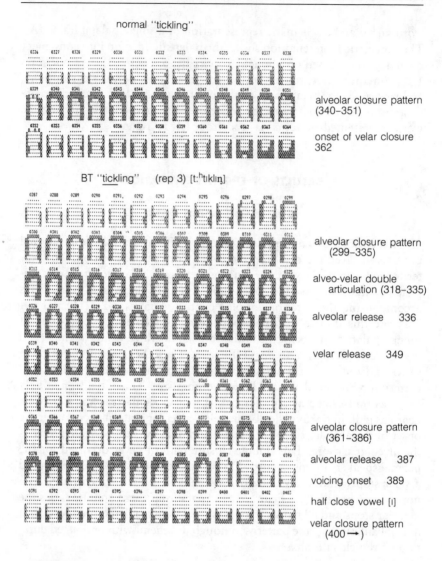

normal "tickling"

alveolar closure pattern (340–351)

onset of velar closure 362

BT "tickling"   (rep 3) [t:ʰtɪklɪŋ]

alveolar closure pattern (299–335)

alveo-velar double articulation (318–335)

alveolar release   336

velar release   349

alveolar closure pattern (361–386)

alveolar release   387

voicing onset   389

half close vowel [ɪ]

velar closure pattern (400 →)

FIGURE 7-2. Tongue-palate contacts for the initial stop in *tickling.*

ALVEOLAR FRICATIVE. BT's patterns were within normal limits in most items in both initial and final position. The tongue configuration was quite spread with anterior lateral contact and a relatively wide central groove. The auditory impression was of a normal fricative. One repetition of *zoo* however showed an abnormal onset pattern with a complex series of contacts including an alveolar closure followed by a velar closure (see Figure 7-6). This sequence was transcribed as [dəgzu:]. Notice that the initial alveolar closure was preceded by a velar stop pattern which was not detected auditorily. All other repetitions of *zoo* were produced normally.

normal "deer"

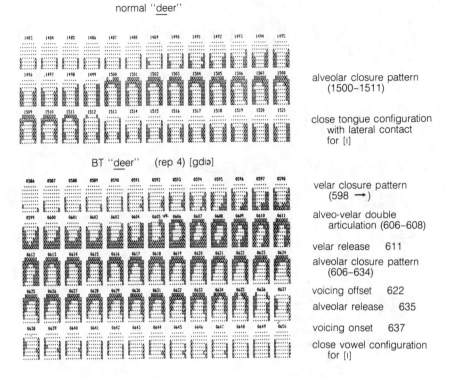

alveolar closure pattern
(1500–1511)

close tongue configuration
with lateral contact
for [ɪ]

BT "deer"   (rep 4) [gdɪə]

velar closure pattern
(598 →)

alveo-velar double
articulation (606–608)

velar release   611
alveolar closure pattern
(606–634)

voicing offset   622

alveolar release   635

voicing onset   637

close vowel configuration
for [ɪ]

FIGURE 7-3. Tongue-palate contacts for the initial stop in *deer*.

PLATO ALVEOLAR FRICATIVE. Inconsistent patterns occurred in word initial position. The most common pattern produced by BT was an /s/-type onset followed immediately by a palatal grooved configuration characteristic of BT's normal /ʃ/ pattern (see Figure 7-7 for *shop*). Occasionally the /s/ substitution pattern remained uncorrected (e.g., in two repetitions of *sheep*, see Figure 7-8). Other variant productions included an intrusive /p/ detected auditorily after an initial /s/ and a velar stop pattern initiating the fricative pattern in one repetition of "shark". The intrusive velar stop pattern occurred also in one repetition of *sheep* (Figure 7-9) where a complete alveolar stop pattern was followed almost immediately by a velar stop giving a simultaneous alveolar/velar closure. The transcription was given as [s:>ʃɪp] indicating that the velar pattern remained undetected auditorily. The variability in patterns produced on successive repetitions of the same word is particularly noticeable in three repetitions of *shark* (Figure 7-10).

Data on Consonant Sequences

STOP-STOP SEQUENCES (/tk, kt, kd/). In producing these sequences, BT showed variable patterns with some evidence of abnormal sequencing of the velar and alveolar articulatory gestures. In a number of cases the

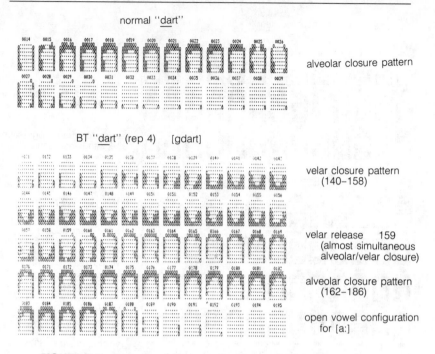

normal "dart"

alveolar closure pattern

BT "dart" (rep 4)   [gdart]

velar closure pattern
(140–158)

velar release   159
(almost simultaneous
alveolar/velar closure)

alveolar closure pattern
(162–186)

open vowel configuration
for [a:]

FIGURE 7-4. Tongue-palate contacts for the initial stop in *dart*.

disordered sequence showed evidence of metathesis. For example in *catkin* the ordering of the /tk/ sequence was reversed (see Figure 7-11). In other items there was difficulty in achieving a smooth transition between the two elements in the consonant sequence. This could be interpreted in some cases as the lack of normal anticipatory coarticulation. For example in the /kd/ sequence in *weekday* there was clear evidence in the EPG print-out of the velar stop being released before movement upwards and for-wards for the alveolar /d/ element. Normal patterns would show the coar-ticulatory effect with a double articulation pattern involving simultaneous velar and alveolar closure. The lack of smooth transition was seen also in other clusters involving stops (e.g., the /kl/, /dl/ sequences) and may be a simplifying strategy adopted by BT to facilitate the sequential manipulations of the tongue-body and tongue-tip-blade system required for these juxtaposed elements.

STOP-FRICATIVE AND FRICATIVE-STOP SEQUENCES (/ts, ks, kʃ, sk, st, ʃk/. As was the case when produced as a single consonant, BT's /ʃ/ showed con-siderable variability in clusters sometimes being produced with the /s/-like onset. The sequences /ks/, /sk/, and /st/ were in general produced nor-mally but all four repetitions of /ts/ as in *hats* showed consistent velar stop patterns instead of the target alveolar (heard as [hæks]).

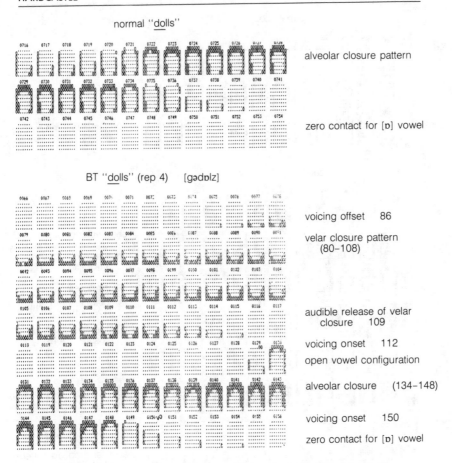

FIGURE 7-5. Tongue-palate contacts for the initial stop in *dolls*.

FRICATIVE-LATERAL AND LATERAL-FRICATIVE SEQUENCES (/sl, ʃl, lʃ, ls/).
BT's EPG patterns for these sequences were in general normal and they
were perceived also as normal. The exceptions were some attempts at /ʃ/
which has an /s/-like onset (see above) and /ʃl/ had abnormal timing
patterns.

STOP-LATERAL SEQUENCES (/dl, kl/). BT showed consistently abnormal
timing patterns in these sequences including the release of the /k/ closure
well prior to the onset of the /l/ in *clock* (170 ms compared to normal
maximum 30 ms, see Figure 7-12) and an abnormally long closure phase
for all repetitions of the /d/ in *headlight*. In all cases the spatial patterns
were normal in every respect.

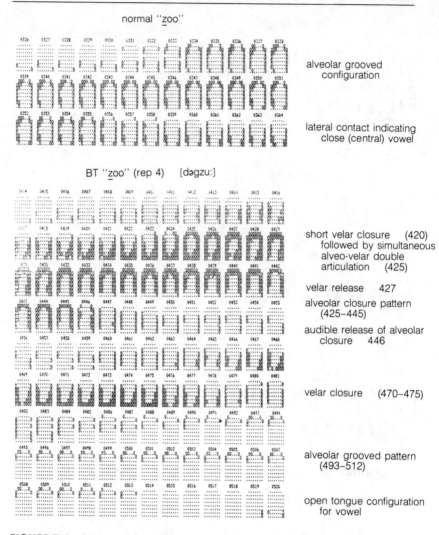

FIGURE 7-6. Tongue-palate contacts for the initial fricative in *zoo*. Note that the velar onset (420–425) was undetected auditorily.

DISCUSSION

Observation of BT's tongue contact patterns revealed a number of general tendencies. Firstly the patterns were markedly variable, not only for repetitions of the same phoneme target in different environments but for successive repetitions of the same word (e.g., the EPG patterns for three repetitions of *shark*, Figure 7-10). The variability of errors has traditionally been seen as one of the hallmarks of dyspraxic speech and helps to

normal "shop"

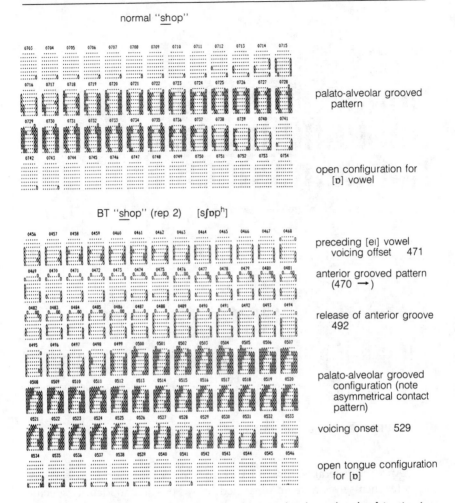

palato-alveolar grooved pattern

open configuration for [ɒ] vowel

BT "shop" (rep 2)   [sʃɒpʰ]

preceding [eɪ] vowel
voicing offset   471

anterior grooved pattern
(470 →)

release of anterior groove
492

palato-alveolar grooved
configuration (note
asymmetrical contact
pattern)

voicing onset   529

open tongue configuration
for [ɒ]

FIGURE 7-7. Tongue-palate contacts for the initial palato-alveolar fricative in *shop*.

differentiate it from most dysarthrias, where the errors are relatively more predictable (e.g., compare EPG patterns for dyspraxic and dysarthric speech in Hardcastle et al., 1985). As Rosenbek and colleagues (1984) suggest: "Our clinical rule is that dysarthria is the most likely diagnosis if a patient has a high proportion of relatively consistent distortions. Apraxia of speech is the likely diagnosis if distortions are mixed with what sound like substitutions especially if such errors are relatively inconsistent."

The errors tended to occur in word initial position. This tendency also has been noted by other investigators and has been interpreted as reflecting the relatively more complex motor encoding required for this position (e.g., Kent & Rosenbek, 1983).

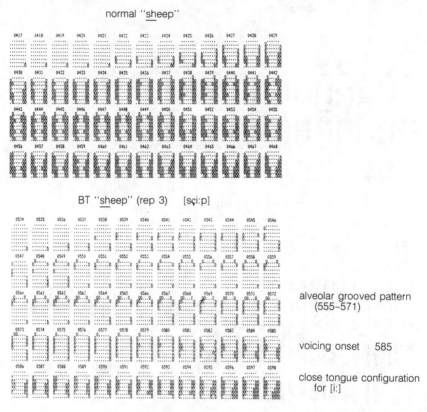

FIGURE 7-8. Tongue-palate contacts for the initial fricative in *sheep*.

Another general feature of BT's error patterns is that the articulatory gestures themselves were not distorted. It was possible to identify specific component gestures in the complex sequence of patterns produced by BT, including, for example, a velar closure gesture, an alveolar closure gesture, an alveolar grooved gesture, and a palato–alveolar grooved gesture. All these component gestures as produced by BT were perfectly normal and consistent as far as their spatial configurations on the palate were concerned and could be readily identified even during the auditorily detected errors. Thus the velar closure gesture occurred simultaneously with the alveolar closure gesture in the double articulation pattern perceived as a "distorted" [d] at the onset of *deer* (Figure 7-3), and the alveolar grooved gesture occurred just prior to the correct target palato-alveolar gesture in *sheep* (Figure 7-8). Even in the most complex errors, such as the initial sequence in *zoo* (Figure 7-6), these component gestures could be identified from the EPG patterns. The component gestures were thus normal spatially; what was disturbed was their temporal integration and their occurrence at inappropriate places.

normal "sheep"

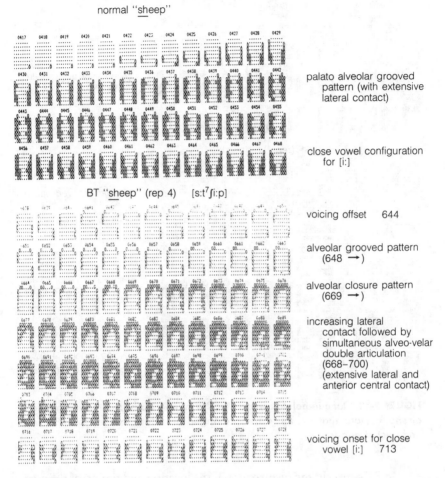

palato alveolar grooved
pattern (with extensive
lateral contact)

close vowel configuration
for [i:]

BT "sheep" (rep 4)   [s:t⁷ʃi:p]

voicing offset   644

alveolar grooved pattern
(648 →)

alveolar closure pattern
(669 →)

increasing lateral
contact followed by
simultaneous alveo-velar
double articulation
(668–700)
(extensive lateral and
anterior central contact)

voicing onset for close
vowel [i:]   713

FIGURE 7-9. Tongue-palate contacts for the initial fricative in *sheep*. Note that the velar closure was not detected auditorily.

The situation is quite different in the dysarthrias where the gestures themselves show clear evidence of "true" distortion, for example, partial alveolar closure (undershoot) rather than full alveolar closure, which reflects inappropriate muscular control (see Hardcastle et al., 1985). What is important in the present context is that even though many of the errors made by BT were perceived (and transcribed as) phonetic distortions, for example, the initial stop in *deer* heard as an abnormal [d], the component gestures involved—namely the alveolar and velar closure gestures—were quite normal in themselves and, in fact, characterized both BT's and the normal speaker's production of the phonemes /d/ and /g/ respectively.

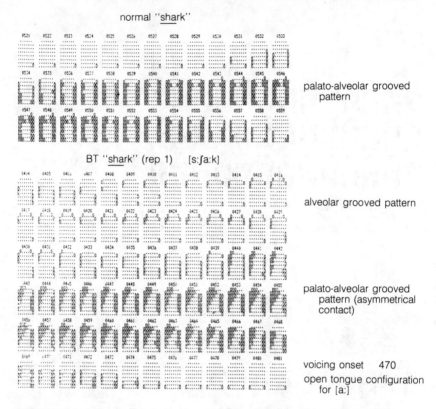

FIGURE 7-10. Tongue-palate contacts for the initial fricatives in three repetitions of *shark*. Note that in rep. 4 the prolonged alveolar closure (456–489) was undetected auditorily.

In BT's speech, the disturbance in the location and timing of the component articulatory gestures often led to stuttering-like symptoms. The so-called core components of stuttering—elemental repetitions and prolongations (Wingate, 1964)—occurred frequently. The prolongations involved nasals (e.g., *milking* as [m:ɪəkɪn]), fricatives (e.g., *shop* as [s:s:sʃapʰ]), as well as the closure phases of stops (e.g., *tickling*, as in Figure 7-2). Repetitions involving syllables or monosyllabic words occurred, but usually, unlike in ideopathic stuttering, only one repetition was produced and this involved either the target syllable itself or a syllable similar to the target except for the final segment. Thus [eɪ lɛg lɛg], [eɪ lɛd lɛg] and [ə li:k li:f]. In all cases where the first attempt at the target word was incorrect, a real word was, in fact, produced rather than a neologism. This may perhaps reflect a mild lexical selection problem in this patient. Elemental repetitions of CV sequences occurred also and here the vowel was similar both perceptually and in terms of contact pattern to the target vowel (cf. elemental repetitions

BT "shark" (rep 2)   [s.ʃaːk]

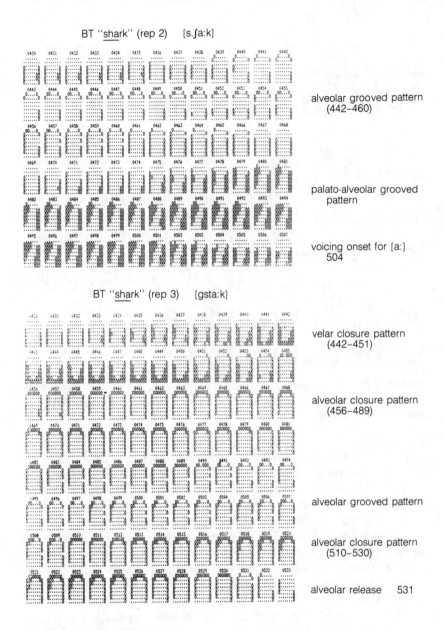

alveolar grooved pattern
(442-460)

palato-alveolar grooved
pattern

voicing onset for [aː]
504

BT "shark" (rep 3)   [gstaːk]

velar closure pattern
(442-451)

alveolar closure pattern
(456-489)

alveolar grooved pattern

alveolar closure pattern
(510-530)

alveolar release   531

FIGURE 7-10 (continued).

129

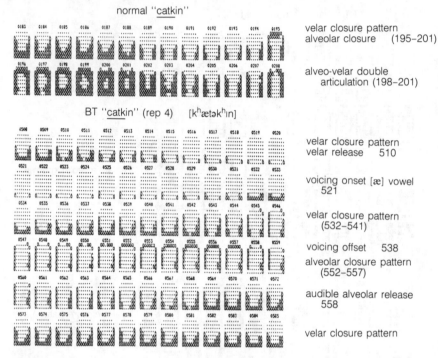

FIGURE 7-11. Tongue-palate contacts for the intervocalic consonant sequence /tk/ in the word *catkin*. Note that the second velar closure (532–541) was undetected auditorily.

in ideopathic stuttering where, according to Van Riper (1971), a *schwa*-type vowel usually occurs). The stuttering-like disfluency features have frequently been associated with dyspraxic speech (see e.g., Johns & Darley, 1970; Trost, 1971) and are probably subsumed under the familiar symptoms of dyspraxia: *retrials*, *sound searching*, and *groping*.

Detailed analysis of BT's EPG patterns shows evidence that some sort of ongoing sensory monitoring is being used by this patient. In almost all cases an error is immediately detected, sometimes directly after the onset of an inappropriate articulatory gesture (e.g., 70 ms after the velar closure at the onset of *deer* and *zoo*—Figures 7-3 and 7-6). In cases such as the latter it is probable that tactile or proprioceptive feedback systems are operating in detecting the error. In other cases where there is a release of the initial incorrect gesture (e.g., the velar closure gesture onset of *dolls*— Figure 7-5), auditory cues are available for monitoring and are probably utilized by BT. The prompt detection and correction of the inappropriate articulatory gesture may differentiate the dyspraxic patient from fluent aphasics where, presumably, because of impaired feedback monitoring, the

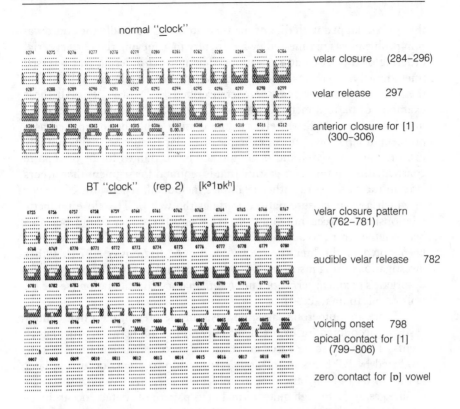

normal "clock"

velar closure   (284-296)

velar release   297

anterior closure for [1]
(300-306)

BT "clock"   (rep 2)   [kᵊ1ɒkʰ]

velar closure pattern
(762-781)

audible velar release   782

voicing onset   798
apical contact for [1]
(799-806)

zero contact for [ɒ] vowel

FIGURE 7-12. Tongue-palate contacts for the /kl/ sequence in the word *clock*.

errors remain largely uncorrected. It is also important to note that the evidence for the rapid ongoing type of monitoring that seems to operate in such cases as *deer* is available only from instrumental analyses, such as EPG, and would not be detected auditorily.

The specific errors produced by BT offer some important clues as to the nature of verbal dyspraxia. There is evidence of both a general articulatory coordination problem and also of a problem in the selection of target gestures. The general coordination problem is manifested in various ways. Firstly there is a problem in achieving smooth transitions between successive articuiatory gestures. This was particularly noticeable in the consonant sequences and frequently involved difficulty in achieving normal anticipatory coarticulation between the tongue tip and blade and the body of the tongue. The typical manifestations were an abnormally long delay from the release of the first element before the onset of the second (as in the /kl, kd, dl, and tk/ clusters). In these cases either the first element was released and heard as a *schwa*-type vowel or the first closure was prolonged. Occasionally, however, normal anticipatory coarticulation occurred as in one repetition of *bookshop* in which the onset of the gesture for the /ʃ/ overlapped with that of the velar stop /k/. Secondly the coordination problem was manifested by a difficulty in achieving the correct serial ordering of the articulatory gestures. The normal ordering was reversed (metathesis) in some /tk, kt/ sequences (e.g., *catkin*—Figure 7-11) and in the /sk/ sequence of *squashkit* (transcribed as [gs ask: ɪtʰ]. All these examples of pattern metathesis involved velars and alveolas. Some of the instances of the intrusive velar closure gesture could be interpreted as a problem in seriation also. For example, the velar closure occurring initially in words such as *shark* and *tickling* could be accounted for by premature coarticulation of the velar gesture that is required for segment that occurs later in the same word (other examples include all repetitions of *tractor* in which a velar closure pattern initiates the word). The close phonetic relationship between not only the error and the target sound but also between the error and another element in the intended word has frequently been noted in the literature (e.g., Martin & Rigrodsky, 1974). Other investigations using instrumental techniques have interpreted many of the dyspraxic's errors in terms of faulty anticipatory coarticulation (see, e.g., Itoh & Sasanuma, 1984).

There are numerous cases, however, in the present data that cannot easily be accounted for by problems in coordination between articulatory events. There are some cases in which the incorrect articulatory gesture produced by BT bears no obvious relationship to events occurring later in the words and appears to be a problem in selection. An intrusive velar closure gesture, although quite normal in its pattern of contact, occurs inappropriately at the onset of one repetition of *deer*, one repetition of *dart* and at the onset of two repetitions of *dolls*, although in the latter case no simultaneous alveolar-velar closure ensues, the velar being released before the alveolar stop. The instrusive velar closure occurs quite frequently in the EPG data but usually remains undetected in the auditory analysis. For example, neither the velar stop onset in *zoo* (Figure 7-5) nor the velar closure component initially in *tickling* (Figure 7-2) or *sheep* (Figure 7-9) were noted in the phonetic transcription of these words.

Other instances of selection errors involve the fricative targets. The palatoalveolar target /ʃ/ is frequently initiated by an /s/-type gesture usually (but not always) corrected, and the required /ʃ/ pattern produced. It is difficult to explain these selection-type errors in terms of a motor coordination problem particularly as the articulatory gestures that are produced in place of the target are in no way distorted and are associated with the production of normal target phonemes elsewhere in BT's utterances. These substituted patterns are usually perceived as being related closely to the target. For example closure gestures (perceived as stop phonemes) replace other stop gestures but at a different place of articulation, fricative patterns replace target fricatives also differing in place. (Thus, target alveolar stops are heard as velar stops, target /ʃ/ is produced as [s]). Occasionally, however, the substituted pattern bears little relationship to the target (see, for example, the complex series of stop- and fricative-type gestures initiating the words *shark* [3rd rep.] and *zoo*—Figures 7-6 and 7-10).

It is clear from the foregoing that a precise description of the speech characteristics of verbal dyspraxia will be extremely difficult, if not impossible, if sole reliance is placed on auditory judgments of the speech output of these patients. In the past impressionistic terms such as "distortions" and "substitutions" have been used to categorize the errors made by such patients, but the use of such terms can be quite misleading. For example, many of the errors made by BT, e.g., the /d/ in *deer*, are heard as distortions of target phonemes; but an analysis of the EPG patterns reveal that such "distortions" come about by various combinations of component articulatory gestures which are in themselves quite normal. It is certainly misleading to use the same term to refer to errors caused by specific neuromuscular impairment resulting in abnormal component articulatory gestures (such as undershoot of component tongue-contact patterns in dysarthric speech).

CONCLUSIONS

The following characteristics of BT's speech were revealed by a detailed analysis of his EPG patterns and the inferred underlying tongue activities:

- Patterns of tongue-palate contact were extremely variable both temporally and spatially not only for the target sound in different environments but for the sound in successive repetitions of the same word.
- Most errors occurred in initial position and in consonant clusters.
- Disfluent symptoms occurred including prolongations and repetitions of monosyllabic words and syllables. The latter differed from the type of repetitions typical of ideopathic stuttering.
- BT's tongue contact patterns could be categorized in terms of four inferred articulatory gestures: an alveolar closure gesture, an alveolar grooved gesture, a palato-alveolar grooved gesture, and a velar closure gesture. These component articulatory gestures were normal in terms of their spatial configuration on the palate and were associated with the production of specific phonemes both in BT's fluent utterances and in the speech of normal subjects. The auditorily detected errors in BT's speech were interpreted in the following ways: (1) selection of an inappropriate articulatory gesture for a specific target phoneme (e.g., [s] for /ʃ/ in *sheep*); (2) incorrect serial ordering of articulatory gestures (e.g., metathesis in *catkin*, intrusive [k] at onset of *shark*); (3) inability to effect smooth

transition between successive articulatory gestures (e.g., delay from
[k] to [l] in *clock*).
• Most inappropriate articulatory gestures were detected and corrected by BT showing evidence of intact sensory feedback monitoring systems.

Many of these features may provide important clues for differential
diagnosis of verbal dyspraxia. For example, the latter would presumably
be relevant for differentiating a dyspraxia from fluent aphasia. In fluent
aphasia one would expect feedback monitoring to be impaired and this
should be reflected in the details of lingual contact patterns. Observation
of the articulatory component gestures mentioned in the Haird
Characteristic would give important clues for distinguishing dyspraxia from
dysarthria as would the consistency of pattern in the first characteristic.
In dysarthria, component gestures would usually be distorted in their spatial
configuration and be more consistently produced. Such instrumental techniques as EPG would seem to offer new insights into the nature of these
disorders, as many of the relevant features mentioned here are not detected
by an auditory based analysis.

ACKNOWLEDGMENTS

Thanks are due to Rosemarie Morgan Barry and Chris Clark for
assistance in carrying out this project and to Susan Edwards and Fiona
Gibbon for helpful comments on the manuscript. The work was supported
by a grant from the British Medical Research Council (Project Grant No.
G8201596N).

REFERENCES

Alfonso, P.J., & Baer, T. (1982). Dynamics of vowel articulation. *Language and
Speech, 15,* 151–173.
Amorosa, H., von Benda, U. Wagner, E., & Keck, A. (1985). Transcribing phonetic
detail in the speech of unintelligible children: A comparison of procedures. *British
Journal of Disorders of Communication, 20,* 281–287.
Blumstein, S. (1973). *A phonological investigation of aphasic speech.* Janua
Linguarum Series Minor 153. The Hague: Mouton.
Blumstein, S., Cooper, W.E., Goodglass, H., Statlender, S., & Gottlieb, J. (1980).
Production deficits in aphasia: A voice-onset time analysis. *Brain and Language,
9,* 153–170.
Darley, F.L. (1967). Lacunae and research approaches to them, IV. In Millikan,
C.H. and Darley, F.L. (Eds.), *Brain mechanisms underlying speech and language.*
New York: Grune & Stratton, pp. 236–290.

Darley, F.L. (1982). *Aphasia*. New York: Saunders.

Deal, J.L., & Darley, F.L. (1972). The influence of linguistic and situational variables on phonemic accuracy in apraxia of speech. *Journal of Speech and Hearing Research, 15*, 639–653.

Duffy, J.R., & Gawle, C.A. (1984). Apraxic speakers' vowel duration in consonant-vowel-consonant syllables. In J.C. Rosenbek, M.R. McNeil, & A.E. Aronson (Eds.), *Apraxia of speech: Physiology, acoustics, linguistics, management*. San Diego: College-Hill Press, pp. 167–196.

Edwards, M. (1984). *Disorders of articulation: Aspects of dysarthria and verbal dyspraxia*. Vienna: Springer.

Hardcastle, W.J. (1984). New methods of profiling lingual palatal contact patterns with electropalatography. *Phonetics Laboratory of the University of Reading Work in Progress, 4*, 1–40.

Hardcastle, W.J., Morgan Barry, R.A., & Clark, C.J. (1985). Articulatory and voicing characteristics of adult dysarthric and verbal dyspraxic speakers: an instrumental study. British Journal of Disorders of Communication, 20, 249–270.

Hardcastle. W.J., Morgan Barry, R.A., & Clark, C.J. (1987). An instrumental phonetic study of lingual activity in articulation-disordered children. *Journal of Speech & Hearing Research* (In Press).

Itoh, M., & Sasanuma, S. (1984). Articulatory movement in apraxia of speech. In J.C. Rosenbek, M.R. McNeil, & A.E. Aronson (Eds.). *Apraxia of speech: Physiology, acoustics, linguistics, management*. San Diego: College Hill Press, pp. 135–166.

Johns, D.F., & Darley, F.L. (1970). Phonemic variability in apraxia of speech. *Journal of Speech and Hearing Research, 13*, 556–583.

Kent, R.D. & Rosenbek, J.C. (1983). Acoustic patterns of apraxia of speech. *Journal of Speech and Hearing Research, 26*, 231–249.

Lesser, R. (1978). *Linguistic Investigations of Aphasia*. London: Edward Arnold.

Martin, A.D., & Rigrodsky, S. (1974). An investigation of phonological impairment in aphasia. *Cortex, 10*, 317–328.

Miyawaki, K. (1974). A study of the musculature of the human tongue (observations on transparent preparations of serial sections). Annual Bulletin, Research Institute of Logopedics and Phoniatrics, University of Tokyo 8, 23–50.

Rosenbek, J.C., Kent, R.D., & La Pointe, L.L. (1984). Apraxia of speech: An overview and some perspectives. In J.C. Rosenbek, M.R. McNeil, & A.E. Aronson (Eds.), *Apraxia of speech: Physiology, acoustics, linguistics, management*. San Diego: College-Hill Press, pp. 1–72.

Rosenbek, J.C., McNeil, M.R., & Aronson, A.E. (1984). *Apraxia of speech, physiology, acoustics, linguistics, management*. San Diego: College-Hill Press.

Trost, J.E. (1971). Apraxic disfluency in patients with Broca's aphasia (Paper presented at the American Speech and Hearing Association Convention, Chicago).

Trost, J., & Canter, C. (1974). Apraxia of speech in patients with Broca's aphasia. *Brain and Language, 1*, 63–80.

Van Riper, C. (1971). *The nature of stuttering*. Englewood Cliffs, NJ: Prentice-Hall.

Wingate, M.E. (1964) A standard definition of stuttering. *Journal of Speech and Hearing Disorders 29*, 484–489.

APPENDIX 7-1

Words used as test items in the measurement of lingual-palatal contact patterns. Lists A and B are used to elicit single lingual consonant sounds (d, t, k, g, l, n, s, z, ʃ, tʃ) in a variety of environments, and list C elicits consonant sequences both within a single morpheme and across morpheme boundaries. All items are illustrated on flash cards that display both the written word and a pictorial representation. In all cases, where grammatically appropriate, the item is preceded by the definite or indefinite article.

List A	*List B*	*List C*
a dart	a sun	the salt
a lamb	a mouse	a KitKat
a cot	a fish	a headlight
a deer	a zoo	a clock
a leg	a sheep	a tractor
a chain	a brush	the Hulk
a shark	a seed	a catkin
a key	a shop	a milking
the dolls	a bush	a weekday
a leaf	a shoe	a tickling
a book	a racer	a deckchair
a well		a bookshop
a car		a Welsh
a girl		a star
a beak		a crashlanding
a knot		a box
		a slide
		a bikeshop
		a fishcake
		the hats
		a squashkit
		a skirt
		the fish soup

Articulatory Velocities of Aphasic Patients

Motonobu Itoh
Sumiko Sasanuma

Ever since the era of Broca and Wernicke, differences in the speech patterns of anterior and posterior aphasic patients have been recognized. Among other things, slowness of articulation in anterior aphasic patients has been emphasized by many clinicians and researchers and considered an important factor in these patients' nonfluent speech. Such an observation, however, is usually based on perceptual evaluation (listener's impression), calculation of speaking rate (counting the number of utterances in a given unit), or, at best, spectrographic measurement of durations. Even the last method is indirect and its results are sometimes misleading. We have pointed out the limitations of durational measurements as a method of estimating articulatory speed elsewhere (Itoh et al., 1980).

We believe that articulatory velocity data are important for determining whether motor deficits exist in anterior aphasic patients and that it is imperative to directly measure the articulatory speed of aphasic patients to determine whether anterior aphasic patients move their articulators more slowly than posterior aphasic patients do. Thus, we attempted to collect velocity and displacement data for labial and mandibular articulatory movements in different phonetic contexts from both Broca's and Wernicke's aphasic patients making use of a photo-optical instrument that consisted of a position-sensitive device and light emitting diodes.

METHOD

Subjects

The experimental subjects were 5 Broca's and 3 Wernicke's aphasic patients of the Tokyo Metropolitan Geriatric Hospital. Table 8-1 shows

TABLE 8-1. *Experimental Subjects*

Site of Lesion	Age	Sex	Aphasia Type	Aphasia Severity	POm* (months)
Anterior	50	F	Broca	Mild	13
	55	M	Broca	Mild	28
	61	M	Broca	Mild	17
	62	M	Broca	Mild–moderate	23
	49	M	Broca	Moderate	16
Posterior	53	F	Wernicke	Mild	94
	68	M	Wernicke	Mild–moderate	10
	47	M	Wernicke	Mild–moderate	39

*Post-Onset time.

their age, sex, type and severity of aphasia, and their post-onset time in months. The severity of the aphasic impairment of these patients was mild to moderate. The etiology of each patient was a single cerebrovascular accident, and the site of lesion in every case was determined by CT scan. Ten subjects with normal speech and hearing served as controls. These subjects included both staff members of the Tokyo Metropolitan Institute of Gerontology and volunteers from local senior-citizens groups. Their ages ranged from 20 to 76 years (Table 8-2).

Procedure

As Figure 8-1 shows, two infrared, light-emitting diodes (LEDs) were placed on the center of the upper and lower lips of each subject to observe lip movements. In order to measure lower jaw movements, two other LEDs

TABLE 8-2. *Control Subjects*

	Subject	Age	Sex
Young	YN1	41	M
	YN2	35	M
	YN3	28	F
	YN4	20	F
Aged	AN1	71	M
	AN2	76	M
	AN3	74	M
	AN4	73	F
	AN5	72	F
	AN6	70	F

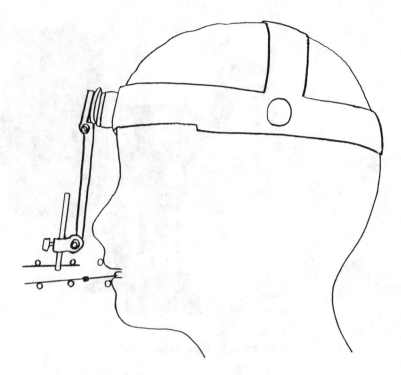

FIGURE. 8-1. Positions of LED

were attached to a solid steel wire that was connected to a lower incisor by means of a resin-splint and a brass wire, which protruded from the gap between the lips. Two additional LEDs were attached to the arm of a head band to monitor the movement of the head. Figure 8-2 shows the experimental set-up. An optical-spot position sensitive detector (PSD) was placed within a camera body, and the image of the LED was focused on the PSD through the camera lens. The distance between the LEDs and the PSD was about 50 cm.

Speech Materials

We prepared three kinds of speech materials: VCV words, sentences, and nonsense monosyllables (Table 8-3). The VCV words consisted of /a/ or /i/ surrounding a nasal(/m/), a stop(/p/or/b/), or a fricative(/s/ or /z/). All of the VCV words were embedded in the carrier phrase - - - *desu* (it is - - -), with stress placed on the second vowel. Each of the VCV words in the carrier phrase were repeated three times in succession. For example, for the word /ama/, the subjects produced /ama desu, ama desu, ama desu/. The data for the second utterance in the sequence was used for analysis. Five data were collected for each of the 16 VCV words, resulting in a total

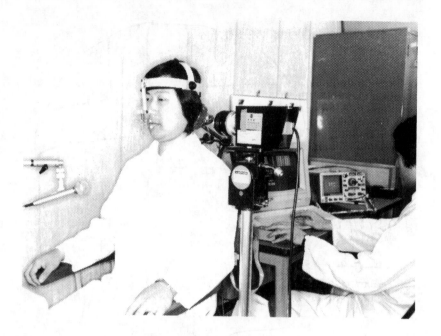

FIGURE 8-2. Experimental set-up

of 80 utterances. The sentences consisted of different numbers of words containing the same word, /yama/, meaning *mountain*. For each of the sentences, three data were obtained, resulting in a total of 15 utterances.

The nonsense monosyllables were /ma/ and /pa/. The subjects were requested to read these speech materials, except the nonsense monosyllables, at a conversational rate, which was demonstrated by the experimenter. For the nonsense monosyllables, the subjects were twice asked to produce as many of each as fast as possible in one breath, and the faster of the two utterance was analyzed.

Analysis of Data

Figure 8-3A shows an example of a side view of the lower lip movement for /ama desu/, and Figure 8-3B shows the time function of the movements along with their audio envelope signal. Point A in each figure indicates the point of the maximum lip opening for the first vowel /a/, and B indicates the point of the maximum lip closing for the consonant /m/. C marks the point of the maximum lip opening for the second vowel /a/.

The displacement magnitude was defined as the distance between points A and B, and between B and C, in the top figure.

TABLE 8-3. *Speech Materials*

/VcV/ words in the frame - - - *desu*

/apa/	/ama/	/imi/	/ima/
/apa/	/api/	/ipi/	/ipa/
/aba/	/abi/	/ibi/	/iba/
/asa/			/isa/
/aza/			/iza/

Sentences
yama desu
yama no e desu
yama no ehagaki desu
    takai *yama* desu
    itibaN takai *yama* desu

Monosyllables
/ma/
/pa/

In order to obtain the maximum velocity, that is, the peak velocity, calculation of the slope of the displacement curve was performed at each data point between A and B, and between B and C, using the seven successive data points of the displacement curve and the method of least squares, with the help of a computer (VAX 11–730). Since the slope of the curve was considered to represent the velocity, the maximum velocity could be defined as the steepest slope. Point D in (B) represents the moment at which the articulator showed its maximum velocity between points A and B, and point E represents that between points B and C.

In a similar way, the displacement and peak velocity of the upper and lower lips and the lower jaw for the other VCV words were measured. The displacement and peak velocity of the VCV portion of the meaningful word /yama/ in the sentences and of the repetitions of /ma/ and /pa/ were also measured in a similar way.

A preliminary analysis of the data has indicated that the data of the lower lip were more informative than those of the upper lip. Therefore, only the results of the lower lip and the lower jaw are reported below.

RESULTS

/VCV/ Words

Figures 8-4 and 8-5 show scatterplots of the lower-lip peak velocity relative to the lower-lip displacement in the /VmV/ words for each of 4 young and 6 aged normal subjects, respectively. The abscissa is the

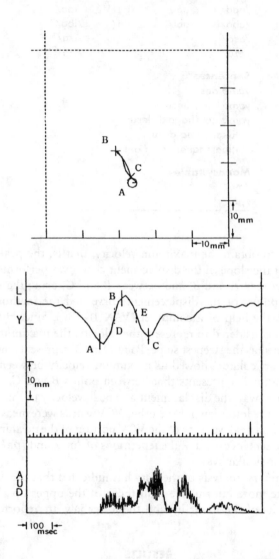

FIGURE 8-3. A side view of lower-lip movement (A) and an example of the time functions of lower-lip movement, along with their audio envelope signal(B) for /ama desu/.

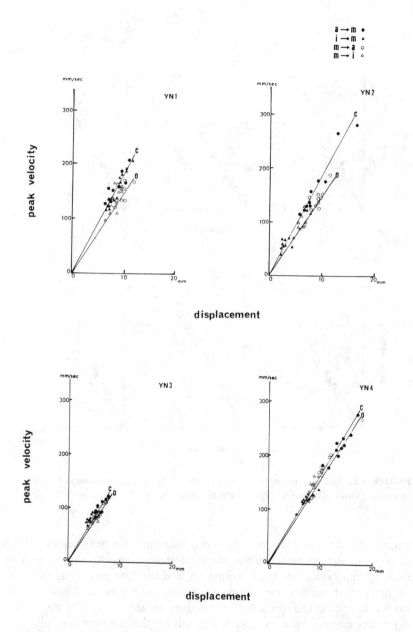

FIGURE 8-4. Scatterplots of B lower-lip peak velocity relative to lower-lip displacement in /VmV/ words for young normal subjects.

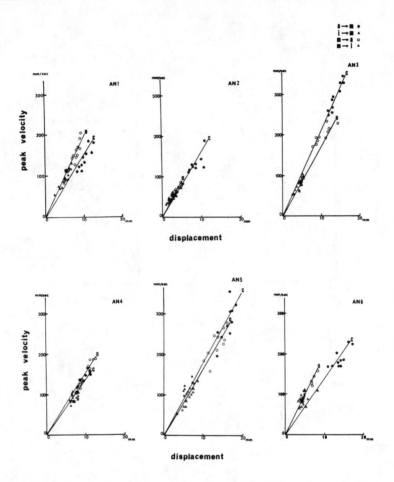

FIGURE 8-5. Scatterplots of lower-lip peak velocity relative to lower-lip displacement in /VmV/ words for aged normal subjects.

magnitude of the displacement, and the ordinate is the peak velocity. The data points for the vowel to the nasal /m/ transition, the closing transition, are represented by the filled marks, and the data points for the /m/ to the vowel transition, the opening transition, are represented by the open marks. In each graph, the subjects' numbers are indicated. YN stands for the young normal subjects, and AN stands for the aged normal subjects. The straight lines shown in each graph were drawn by visual inspection. More specifically, these lines were fitted separately for the closing and opening transition data points and were converged at the origin of the coordinate axes.

It can be observed that these data points fit well with each closing and opening transition line, and that the peak velocity has a strong positive correlation with the magnitude of the displacement. This result suggests that the peak velocity increases with an increase in the displacement of the lower lip, with the time that takes the articulator to move a certain distance kept constant. There were no age or sex differences among the normal subjects in terms of this trend.

Three out of the 10 normal subjects (YN1, YN2, AN3) showed a steeper slope of line for the closing data points, and two (AN1, AN6) showed a steeper slope of line for the opening data points. The remaining 5 (YN3, YN4, AN2, AN4, AN5) showed no difference between these two lines.

It can also be observed that there are noticeable individual differences in the range of the scatterplots. Similar trends found in the performance for /VmV/ words were observed for /VpV/ and /VbV/ words. It was also found that each subject showed quite similar patterns of performance for the three kinds of /VCV/ words with only a few exceptions.

Figure 8-6 shows scatterplots of the lower lip peak velocity relative to the lower lip displacement in the /VmV/ words for the 5 subjects with Broca's aphasia. In each graph, the subject's numbers are indicated. It can be seen that the peak velocity has a positive correlation with the magnitude of the displacement in the Broca's aphasic patients too, even though the range of each patient's scatterplots is larger than that of the normal subjects. This result suggests that, in general, these patients keep the time in which the articulator moves a certain distance constant, and that their articulatory speed is *not* generally slow.

As can be seen, however, the performance of two patients with Broca's aphasia (B1, B5) was characterized by extremely large values in peak velocity and displacement for some utterances, circled by a solid line, compared to the performance of the normal subjects. Another Broca's aphasic patient (B2) showed an extremely slow peak velocity in some utterances , which is circled by a dotted line.

Three Broca's aphasic patients (B1, B2, B5) showed the same characteristics in /VpV/ and /VbV/ words as observed in /VmV/ words. Figure 8-7 shows the results of the three Wernicke's aphasic subjects for the /VmV/ words, which are close to those of the normal subjects in Figures 8-4 and 8-5. This trend was also observed for /VpV/ and /VbV/ words.

/VsV/, /VzV/ Words

Figures 8-8 and 8-9 show scatterplots of the lower jaw peak velocity relative to the lower jaw displacement in the /VsV/ and /VzV/ words for the young and aged normal subjects, respectively. The velocity and displacement data for the lower jaw were obtained from the 8 normal subjects. The majority of the subjects showed some slowness in the closing transition for certain utterances, as well as extremely restricted magnitudes of both peak velocity and displacement for certain utterances. Figure 8-10

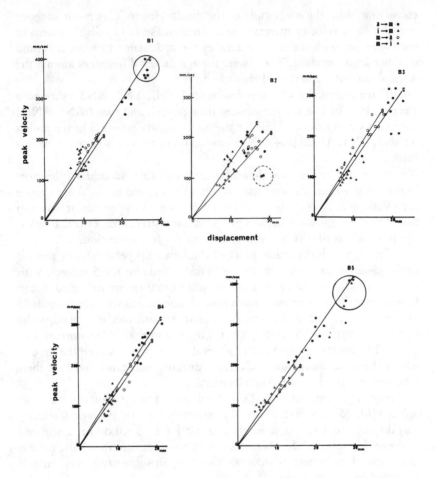

FIGURE 8-6. Scatterplots of lower-lip peak velocity relative to lower-lip displacement in /VmV/ words for Broca's aphasic subjects.

shows scatterplots of the lower-jaw peak velocity relative to the lower jaw displacement in the /VsV/ and /VzV/ words for the patients with Broca's aphasia. The differences in peak velocity between the opening and closing transitions are quite apparent, and the performance of the 4 Broca's aphasic patients (B2, B3, B4, B5) is characterized by an extreme slowness in the closing transition for some utterances, which are indicated by dotted circles or ellipses.

Figure 8-11 shows scatterplots of the lower jaw peak velocity relative to the lower jaw displacement in the /VsV/ and /VzV/ words for two of the patients with Wernicke's aphasia. Both of these patients showed patterns of performance similar to those of the normal subjects.

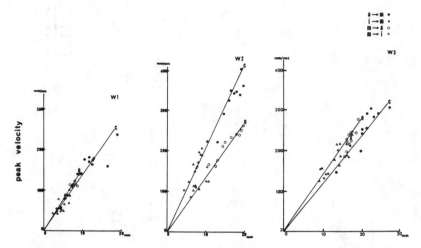

FIGURE 8-7. Scatterplots of lower-lip peak velocity relative to lower-lip displacement in /VmV/ words for Wernicke's aphasic subjects.

/VmV/ in Sentences

Figures 8-12 and 8-13 indicate scatterplots of the lower-lip peak velocity relative to the lower-lip displacement for the /VmV/ portion of the meaningful word /yama/ in the different sentences in the young and aged normal subjects, respectively. It can be seen from these figures that compared with the performance for VmV words in isolation shown in Figures 8-4 and 8-5, variation in both peak velocity and displacement is smaller, resulting in a smaller range of scatterplots, with one exception (YN3), which exhibited a very restricted range of scatterplots for all of the speech materials in the present study.

There was no clear-cut trend for the effect of sentence length and the location of the target (analyzed) word /yama/ in each sentence on the peak velocity.

Figure 8-14 shows scatterplots of the lower-lip peak velocity relative to the lower lip displacement for the /VmV/ portions of the meaningful word /yama/ in the different sentences for the patients with Broca's aphasia. One Broca's aphasic patient (B3) exhibited an extremely slow lower-lip peak velocity in some utterances, indicated by a dotted circle. Interestingly, the majority of these utterances with an extremely slow peak velocity were the long sentences /takai yama desu/ and /itibaN takai yama desu/, in which the target word /yama/ was preceded by other words. The somewhat deviated performance in terms of peak velocity and displacement found in another patient (B5) appears to also be related to sentence length and the location of the target word. It was also observed for the Broca's aphasic

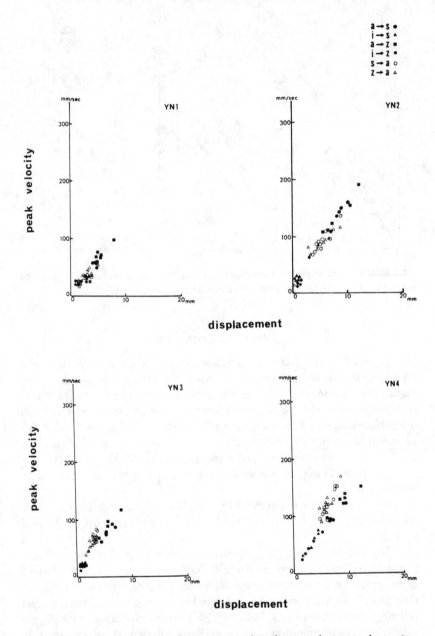

FIGURE 8-8. Scatterplots of lower-jaw peak velocity relative to lower-jaw displacement in the /VsV/ and /VzV/ words for young normal subjects.

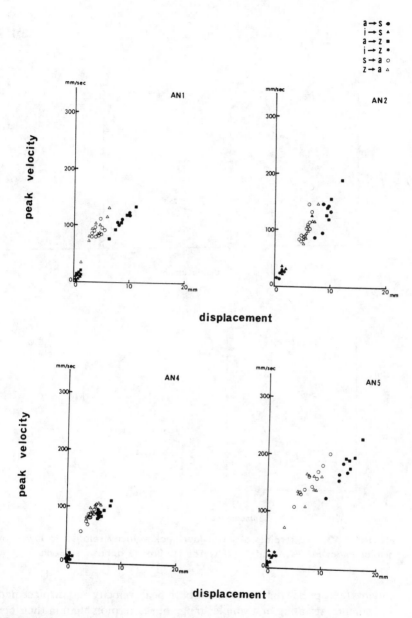

FIGURE 8-9. Scatterplots of lower-jaw peak velocity relative to lower-jaw displacement in /VsV/ and /VzV/ words for aged normal subjects.

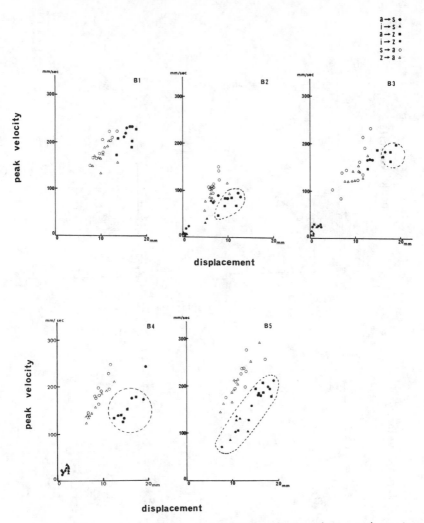

FIGURE 8-10. Scatterplots of lower-jaw peak velocity relative to lower-jaw displacement in /VsV/ and /VzV/ words for Broca's aphasic subjects.

patients (except B3) that variation in both peak velocity and displacement was smaller, resulting in a smaller range of scatterplots than in their performance of /VmV/ words in isolation.

Figure 8-15 shows scatterplots of the lower-lip peak velocity relative to the lower-lip displacement for the /VmV/ portion of the meaningful word /yama/ in the sentences for the three Wernicke's aphasic patients. The range of scatterplots is smaller than that for /VmV/ words in isolation in this group of patients, too.

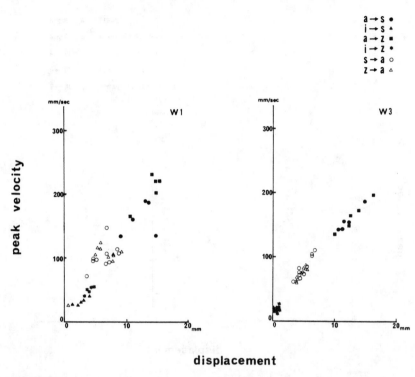

FIGURE 8-11. Scatterplots of lower-jaw peak velocity relative to lower-jaw displacement in /VsV/ and /VzV/ words for Wernicke's aphasic subjects.

/VmV/, /VpV/ in Syllable Repetition

Figures 8-16 and 8-17 present scatterplots of the lower lip peak velocity relative to the lower lip displacement for /VmV/ portions of the repetition of /ma/ in the young and aged normal subjects, respectively. In comparison with /VmV/ words in isolation and sentences, it is apparent that the majority of the normal subjects showed smaller variation in both peak velocity and displacement in the syllable repetition, resulting in the restricted range of the scatterplots. Six out of the 10 subjects (YN2, YN3, YN4, AN1, AN4, AN6) repeated /ma/ with small displacement and relatively low peak velocity of the lower lip, while the remaining 4 subjects (YN1, AN2, AN3, AN5) repeated /ma/ with rather a high peak velocity of the lower lip.

Trends similar to the results for the /VmV/ portions of /ma/ were observed for /VpV/ portions of the repetition of /pa/.

Figures 8-18 and 8-19 show scatterplots of the lower-lip peak velocity relative to the lower-lip displacement for the /VmV/ portions of the

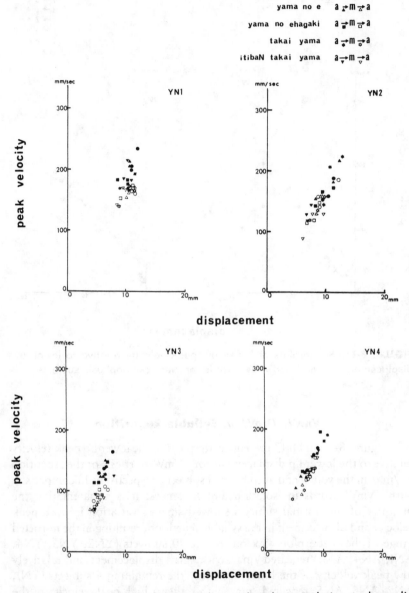

FIGURE 8-12. Scatterplots of lower-lip peak velocity relative to lower-lip displacement in the /(y)ama/ portion of different sentences for young normal subjects.

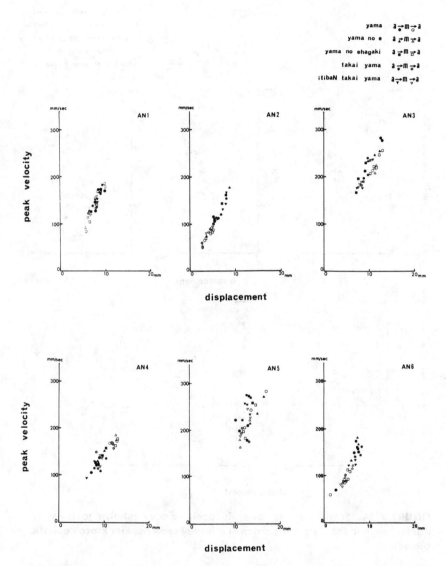

FIGURE 8-13. Scatterplots of lower-lip peak velocity relative to lower-lip displacement in the /(y)ama/ portion of different sentences for aged normal subjects.

153

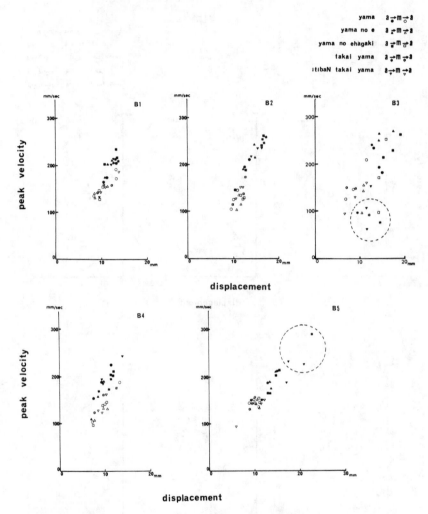

FIGURE 8-14. Scatterplots of lower-lip peak velocity relative to lower-lip displacement in the /(y)ama/ portion of different sentences for Broca's aphasic subjects.

repetition of /ma/ in the Broca's and Wernicke's aphasic patients, respectively.

All of the Broca's and Wernicke's aphasic patients showed patterns of performance similar to those of the normal subjects. Both the Broca's and Wernicke's aphasic patients exhibited similar performance for the /VpV/ portions of the repetition of /pa/. These results indicate that the aphasic patients could normally perform simple, automatic speech tasks such as nonsense monosyllable repetition.

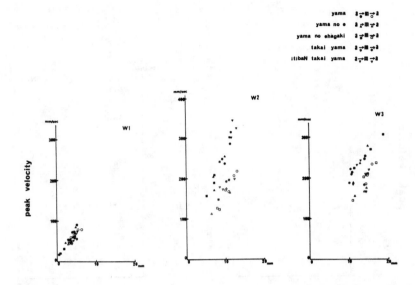

FIGURE 8-15. Scatterplots of lower lip peak velocity relative to lower lip displacement in the /(y)ama/ portion of different sentences for Wernicke's aphasic subjects.

DISCUSSION

It was found that the peak velocity of the articulatory lip and jaw movements had a strong positive correlation with the magnitude of the displacement in various speech productions by normal control subjects. This result suggests that normal speakers keep constant the duration of the articulatory movement for a given phoneme, with a higher peak velocity for a larger displacement of the articulators.

Also, in this study, there were no aberrant changes in terms of articulatory velocity among the aged normal subjects, suggesting that aging does not seem to slow down articulatory speed. This result seems to support the hypothesis that overlearned and frequently performed motor acts, such as speech, are less affected by aging than less frequently performed motor tasks (Kent & Burkard, 1981).

The results for the patients with Broca's aphasia are revealing. Two out of the 5 Broca's aphasic patients showed an extremely high peak velocity, along with an extremely large displacement of the lower lip, in some utterances of /VmV/, /VpV/, and /VbV/ words. Three patients with Broca's aphasia showed an extremely slow lower-lip peak velocity, in spite of a normal magnitude of displacement, for some utterances of /VmV/, /VpV/, and /VbV/ words. Still another Broca's aphasic patient exhibited an

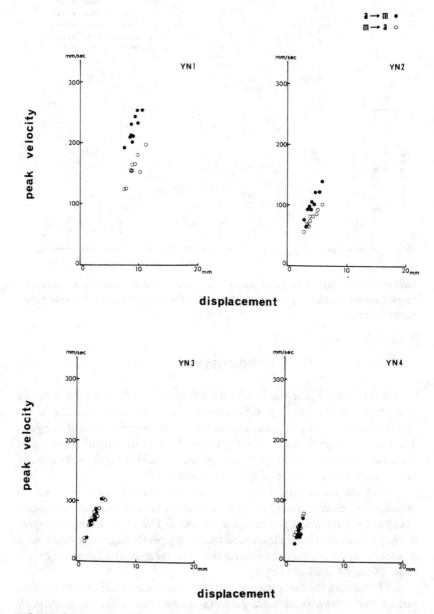

FIGURE 8-16. Scatterplots of lower lip peak velocity relative to lower lip displacement in the /ama/ portion of the repetition of /ma/ for the young normal subjects.

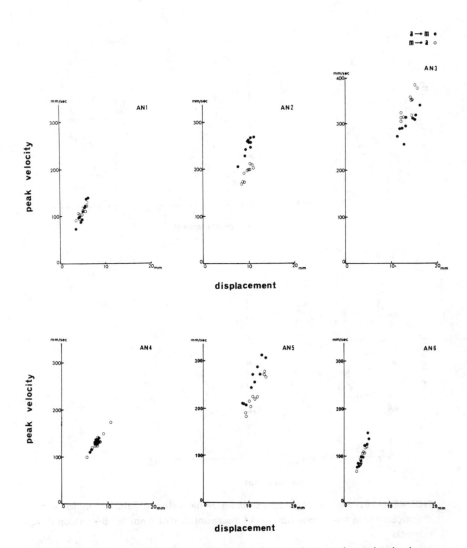

FIGURE 8-17. Scatterplots of lower lip peak velocity relative to lower lip displacement in the /ama/ portion of the repetition of /ma/ for aged normal subjects.

extremely slow peak velocity for some utterances of /(y)ama/ in the longer sentences. This result may have some relationship to the phenomenon that Broca's aphasic patients with apraxia of speech tend to make more errors in longer utterances than in shorter ones (Johns & Darley, 1970). It further suggests that motor programming for speech may become difficult beyond a given length of utterance for some of the patients with Broca's aphasia. In order to examine this assumption, further study is necessary. And finally,

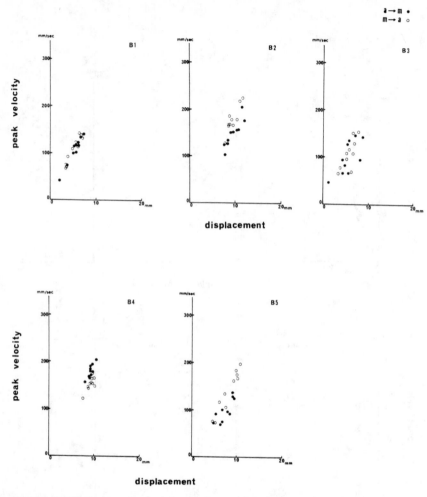

FIGURE 8-18. Scatterplots of lower lip peak velocity relative to lower-lip displacement in the /ama/ portion of the repetition of /ma/ for Broca's aphasic subjects.

the majority of the Broca's aphasic patients exhibited an extremely slow lower-jaw peak velocity in the closing transition for some utterances of the /VsV/ and /VzV/ words. This finding is congruent with the clinical observation that Broca's aphasic patients generally show a conspicuous difficulty in producing fricative sounds (e.g., Johns & Darley, 1970).

It is also important to point out that the speed of the articulators of Broca's aphasic patients is *not* always slow compared to that of normal and Wernicke's aphasic speakers. The performance of Broca's aphasic

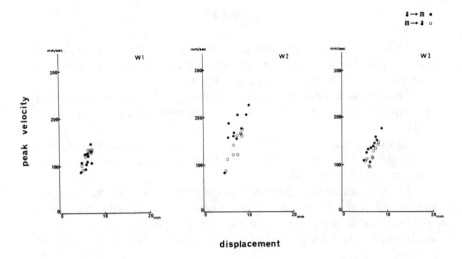

FIGURE 8-19. Scatterplots of lower-lip peak velocity relative to lower-lip displacement in the /ama/ portion of the repetition of /ma/ for Wernicke's aphasic subjects.

patients is rather characterized by inconsistency in terms of articulatory velocity and/or displacement. Coupled with this observation, the finding that the patients with Broca's aphasia do perform normally in the rapid repetition of nonsense monosyllables indicates that their problem is not attributable to paralysis or weakness of the articulatory muscles.

At any rate, the results of the present study indicate that Broca's aphasic patients as a group definitely have difficulty in controlling their articulatory velocity. A disturbance in the control of articulatory velocity will result in a problem with the phasing of individual articulatory gestures, which, in turn, will create difficulties in articulatory transitions, phonetic distortions and dysprosody.

On several occasions, we have pointed out that temporal dyscoordination, and the resultant articulatory and prosodic defects, characterize apraxic speech and can be interpreted as an impairment at the phonetic level of the speech production process (Itoh, Sasanuma, & Ushijima, 1979; Itoh et al., 1980; Itoh et al., 1982; Monoi et al., 1983). We think that this kind of apraxic deficit is an essential component of the speech disturbance in anterior aphasic patients. However, patients with Wernicke's aphasia in our study showed no sign of deviated articulatory behaviors in terms of peak velocity and displacement of the lip and jaw.

All in all, the present study reconfirms our claim that the speech disturbance in anterior aphasic patients reflects an impairment at the phonetic level and can be differentiated from that in posterior aphasic patients (Monoi et al., 1983).

SUMMARY

This study reported the results of an attempt to collect velocity and displacement data for labial and mandibular articulatory movements in both Broca's and Wernicke's aphasic patients.

The data were obtained through a photo-optical instrument consisting of a position sensitive device (PSD) and infrared, light emitting diodes (LED).

As speech materials, 16 VCV (V = a, i; C = p,b,m,s,z) words in a carrier phrase / - - - desu/(it is - - -), 5 sentences, and the monosyllables /ma/ and /pa/ were used.

The displacement magnitude and the peak velocity of the lower-lip and lower-jaw movements in the transitions of V to C and C to V were calculated by a computer based on the displacement curve of each articulator for the VCV portion of each utterance and the method of least squares.

The experimental subjects were 5 Broca's and 3 Wernicke's aphasic patients at the Tokyo Metropolitan Geriatric Hospital and their ages ranged from 47 to 68 years. Six subjects with normal speech and hearing served as controls, and their ages ranged from 20 to 76 years. The major findings were as follows.

First, in the normal control subjects, the peak velocity of the articulatory lip and jaw movements had a strong positive correlation with the magnitude of the displacement. This result suggests that normal speakers keep constant the duration of the articulatory movement for a given phoneme, with a higher peak velocity for a larger displacement of the articulators. Second, there was no aberrant change in articulatory velocity found for the aged normal subjects. Third, the patients with Broca's aphasia exhibited some deviated articulatory behaviors in terms of peak velocity or displacement of the lower lip and the lower jaw. Namely, some patients showed an extremely high peak velocity, along with an extremely large displacement of the lower lip, in some utterances. Other patients showed an extremely slow lower-lip peak velocity, in spite of a normal magnitude of displacement, in some utterances. Additionally, the majority of the Broca aphasic patients exhibited an extremely slow lower-jaw peak velocity in the closing phase of jaw movements in the fricative sound production. These characteristics of the articulatory movements of the patients with Broca's aphasia could be interpreted as constituting one of the important factors contributing to their speech disturbance.

ACKNOWLEDGMENTS

Part of this study was presented at the 20th Congress of the International Association of Logopedics and Phoniatrics held August 3–7, 1986, in Tokyo.

The authors wish to express their sincere thanks to Dr. Shinobu Masaki and Itaru Tatsumi, of the Tokyo Metropolitan Institute of Gerontology, and to Dr. Yoko Fukusako, of the Tokyo Metropolitan Geriatric Hospital, for their cooperation.

REFERENCES

Itoh, M., Sasanuma, S., Hirose, H., Yoshioka, H., & Ushijima, T. (1980). Abnormal articulatory dynamics in a patient with apraxia of speech: X-ray microbeam observation. *Brain and Language*, *11*, 66–75.

Itoh, M., Sasanuma, S., Tatsumi, I.F., Murakami, S., Fukusako, Y., & Suzuki, T. (1982) Voice onset time characteristics in apraxia of speech. *Brain and Language*, *17*, 193–210.

Itoh, M., Sasanuma, S., & Ushijima, T. (1979). Velar movements during speech in a patient with apraxia of speech. *Brain and Language*, *7*, 227–239.

Johns, D., & Darley, F. (1970). Phonemic variability in apraxia of speech. *Journal of Speech and Hearing Research*, *13*, 556–583.

Kent, R.D., & Burkard, R. (1981). Changes in the acoustic correlates of speech production. In D.S. Beasley, and G.A. Davis (Eds.), *Aging: Communication processes and disorders*, New York: Grune & Stratton.

Monoi, H., Fukusako, Y., Itoh, M., & Sasanuma, S. (1983). Speech sound errors in patients with conduction and Broca's aphasia. *Brain and Language*, *20*, 175–194.

Phonetic Realization of Phonological Contrast in Aphasic Patients

Wolfram Ziegler

Aberrations in the sound pattern of aphasic patients are commonly classified into *phonetic* and *phonemic* errors (Blumstein et al., 1977; 1980; Itoh et al., 1982; Tuller, 1984; Hewlett, 1985). Although these labels are descriptive rather than explanatory they are meant to specify the pathomechanism responsible for two distinct error categories: phonemic errors are thought to result from erroneous selection of discrete phonological entities, whereas phonetic errors are ascribed to motor disturbances in the process of their programming or realization. This dichotomy is speculative insofar as it is based upon the constructs of speech production models. Since the two hypothesized stages of the speech production process cannot be examined independently, there is no direct way of assigning any observed instance of an aphasic error to one or the other category.

Nevertheless, some investigators have formulated operational rules, following which a categorization of aphasic errors should be possible. Blumstein and her coworkers investigated aphasic errors of stop-voicing as described by voice-onset time (Blumstein et al., 1977, 1980) and of stop-place of articulation as described by the shape of the burst spectrum (Shinn & Blumstein, 1983)—and used what might be called a *template matching* approach for error classification. Referring to normative data from the literature, they specified fixed ranges of the respective acoustic dimensions (VOT templates or spectral templates) into which correct productions of the considered phonemes should be expected to fall. With a few modifications, phonetic errors were then operationally defined as productions falling between the templates, whereas the productions fitting into an alternative template were termed phonemic errors. An explicit reference to perceptual categories was also made in the error analysis of Shinn & Blumstein (1983).

This classificatory approach has been criticized for its rigidness by several authors (Itoh et al., 1982; Tuller, 1984; Ziegler, 1984; Hewlett, 1985). Blumstein herself stated elsewhere that certain phonological errors "may represent extreme phonetic distortions that are perceived by the listener in terms of a change in phonetic category from the target" (Blumstein, 1981). A differentiation of such aberrations from errors of phonological planning, however, is not captured by a template-fitting criterion. Since phonetic distortions cannot be expected to respect the boundaries of perceptual categories, the application of perceptual reference criteria seems inadequate in a classification of aphasic errors (see Ziegler & Hoole, in press).

In her study on the voicing contrast in initial and final plosives, Tuller (1984) proposed, among other things, a more flexible classification rule that allowed for a shift of the data range describing a patient's productions. She stressed that a delineation of different error types can only be drawn when the overall distribution of acoustic data is bimodal. According to her rule, productions of the voicing distinction are classifiable as phonemic errors when the two modes differ by a certain amount, irrespective of absolute voice onset times. By this rule, however, Tuller introduced another uniform criterion for error classification. The specification of a constant separation interval is strongly language-specific and would require an adjustment when used in languages or dialects in which voicing cognates are separated by shorter or longer VOT intervals (e.g., Lisker & Abramson, 1964). Insisting on a fixed, language-specific relation between voiced and voiceless plosives, however, would imply that an aberration by a certain amount is classified as a phonetic error in one language and as a phonemic error in the other. Itoh et al. (1982) in their VOT study of Japanese aphasics consequently abandonned all uniform threshold criteria and contented themselves with qualitative judgments of VOT distributions in each of their patients. Such a method of considering patterns of phonetic realizations rather than individual instances was also advocated by Hewlett (1985).

The approach presented here starts from a similar view. First, the necessity of distinguishing between at least two different error types is acknowledged. Speech as a purposeful motor act requires the concept of a *plan* for each utterance to be produced. The two opposing members of a minimal pair, for example, can be considered as being represented by two distinct *phonetic plans* (Linnell, 1979) or two different *phonological intentions* (Bromberger & Halle, 1986). Although there might be difficulties in delimiting the physical manifestations of the two contrasting phonetic plans by a clearcut boundary (Fowler, 1985), such plans nevertheless exist as distinct functional goals in the speaker and can be discriminated by the listener. When acoustic or articulatory measures of their realizations are considered statistically, the different goals are recognizable in the emerging bimodal distribution.

A dysfunction in the speech production mechanism may now in principle affect either the discrete structure of phonetic plans or the realization of such plans. A literal paraphasia or phonemic error can in these terms be understood as the realization of an inappropriate phonological intention, i.e., a switch from the adequate target to one of a set of discrete alternatives. A further potential dysfunction at the phonemic level would be the complete breakdown of a feature distinction, meaning that two phonological categories merge. Phonetic errors, on the other hand, arise at one of the subordinate stages of the realization of an—appropriate or inappropriate—phonological intention.

A pervasive phonetic disturbance may cause a not necessarily linear transformation of the phonetic space in which a phoneme opposition is physically manifested. Therefore, both the absolute location of the members of the opposition and their relation to each other may be altered in the considered acoustic or articulatory dimensions. These deviations may attain such an extent that the underlying phonetic plans are no longer identifiable or may appear under the guise of an opposing plan. In individual cases the two potential geneses of aphasic speech errors may therefore lead to physically indistinguishable results. Yet, an analysis of the patient's specific warping of the phonetic space related to a phoneme opposition may help to delineate the two error types.

A formal approach to such an analysis is proposed here. It uses a method of curve fitting to estimate the different components that potentially underlie a distribution of phonetic parameters. The contrastiveness in a great number of realizations of a binary feature is assessed by a parametric model without any assumptions on the particular numerical value of phonetic specifications of the phonological distinction to be made. Using this technique, the two opposing constituents of a binary feature can be considered separately and in relation to each other, the question being whether phonemic unity is preserved in the productions of each of them. Moreover, the realizations of both cognates can be considered in their "lumped distribution," i.e., without any prior knowledge concerning the target to be realized, in order to determine the degree to which phonemic contrast is present.

Most of the applications reported here refer to the voiced–voiceless contrast in plosives as assessed by the acoustic parameter of voice-onset time. An example concerning the rounding contrast in front vowels in terms of formant frequencies is also included.

In a final section the multiple-feature approach proposed by Tuller (1984) is taken up with some modifications. Provided that two independent phonetic cues to one and the same distinctive feature are available, the assumption of a phonemic error would require a categorical change to occur in both underlying phonetic dimensions. If, on the other hand, the two considered parameters do not covary, a phonetic implementation error is more plausible. As an example of such an analysis, the realization of the tense–lax contrast in German vowels as assessed by duration and formant frequency measurements was chosen.

METHODS

Subjects, Materials, and Acoustic Analysis

The aim of this chapter is not so much to describe syndromal differences between aphasic speakers but rather to discuss the methodologicål grounds of a classification of aphasic errors. Therefore, comprehensive case descriptions and correlations with neuroanatomical data are not provided. The data to be described below resulted from different experiments performed with different subjects and different goals. They were obtained from a total of six aphasic patients and an ataxic dysarthric. All patients had suffered from cerebrovascular accidents. Aphasia testing with the Aachener Aphasia Test (AAT) (Huber et al., 1983) revealed a mild Broca's aphasia in A1 and A4, a nonclassifiable aphasia in A2 and A3, and a Wernicke's aphasia in A5 and A6. Patients A1 to A4 had an additional apraxia of speech, the diagnosis of which was based clinically on the presence of substitutions and distortions of speech sounds. All speech apraxics had additional prosodic deficits, i.e., mostly a syllable-by-syllable manner of speaking.

The included subjects were of South German origin. This fact is of some importance in that, unlike Standard German, no voicing lead is to be expected in initial voiced plosives of South German informants.

Patient examinations were based upon different sets of speech material that had in common that they consisted of minimal pairs or near minimal pairs. The pairs differed with respect to initial stop-voicing (/dyCV/ versus /tyCV/, /daCV/ versus /taCV/), to lip rounding (/kɪsən/ (cushion)) versus /kysən/ (to kiss), and to tenseness (/biːtən/ (to offer) versus /bɪtən/ (to request)). Each subject was asked to repeat the stimuli upon aural presentation by an examiner. The target stimuli were separated by a number of dummy words. In no case did the two members of a minimal pair immediately follow each other in the testing. The examinations were run in a sound-treated room and recorded using high quality equipment. Preceding each session the discriminatory abilities of a patient were examined in a same–different task with pairwise aural presentations of the target stimuli described above. All patients included performed well on the auditory discrimination task.

Speech recordings were digitized on a LSI 11/73 for further evaluation. Words containing an error in the target phoneme unrelated to the binary feature under consideration (e.g., a place error in the voiced–voiceless pairs) were excluded from further analysis. Using an interactive routine for display and segmentation of the digitized speech wave, two examiners performed measurements of voice-onset times (VOT) in plosives and of vowel durations following the usual segmentation criteria (e.g., Tuller, 1984). Vowel formants were computed from Linear Predictive Coding (LPC) spectra. The measured data were arranged in histograms using class widths of 10 ms for VOT and vowel durations and of 50 Hz for formant frequencies.

Modeling of Distributions

For each histogram, the number of sampling points was increased by inserting three spline-interpolated points between every two original data points. Figure 9-1 provides an illustration of the procedure to be described in the following. In (A), the figure presents a histogram of VOT values measured for a total of 120 /d/-realizations in /dyCV/ and 120 /t/-realizations in /tyCV/-utterances of a normal subject. Class widths are 10 ms and the frequencies are percentages of N = 240. The vertical bars in (B) indicate interpolated frequencies of occurrence, every fourth bar corresponding to an original value. The solid line represents a model function, which here fits the distribution very closely. Such functions were obtained using a curve-fitting technique with mixed component functions, applied by Scherg & von Cramon (1985) in their dipole model of auditory evoked potentials. In our case we used a class of rational component functions of the form

$$f(t) = \frac{A_o}{(1+(1/b(t-T_o))^2)^2} \quad \text{with} \quad b = \begin{matrix} b_1, t \leq T_o \\ b_r, t > T_o \end{matrix}$$

for curve fitting. These bell-shaped continuous functions assume their maximal value A_o at $t = T_o$ and decrease to $A_o/4$ within the interval $(T_o - b_1, T_o + b_r)$ (see Figure 9-1). The fitting process included determination of the four parameters A_o, T_o, b_1, and b_r such that the sum of squared differences between observed data and approximating function attains a minimum ("least squares fit").

In the one-component approach a single function of the described class was computed with the objective of approximating the empirical data by a unimodal distribution. The two-component approach used a sum of two functions of the earlier-mentioned type as model function, thus identifying two modes that account best for the shape of the considered histogram. The goodness-of-fit of the resulting model was expressed in terms of the *residual variance*, i.e., a quantity measuring the variance of the difference function relative to total variance of the original data.

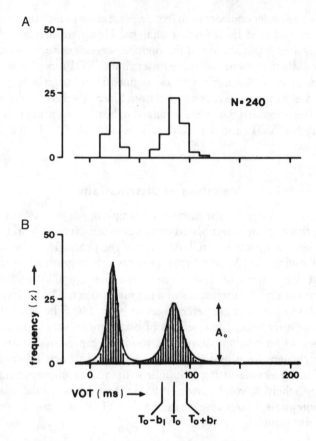

FIGURE 9-1. Distribution of voice onset times of word-initial /d/ and /t/ before /y/ in a normal speaker (N = 240). (A) Relative frequencies of observations within 10 ms classes. (B) Interpolated histogram fitted by a two-component model.

DISCUSSION OF EXAMPLES

Varying Intermodal Distance: Normal and Dysarthric

Figure 9-2 depicts VOT distributions of word-initial /d/ and /t/ in a normal subject (A and B) and an ataxic dysarthric (C). In the bottom panels the data are presented in their lumped distributions, i.e., without any prior grouping of cases. Each histogram was fitted by a one-component model (broken lines) and by a two-component model (solid lines). The resulting residual variances, r_1 and r_2, are specified in the diagrams. In all cases the distributions of single phonemes were almost perfectly described by one-component models. Note that the voiceless plosive always scattered

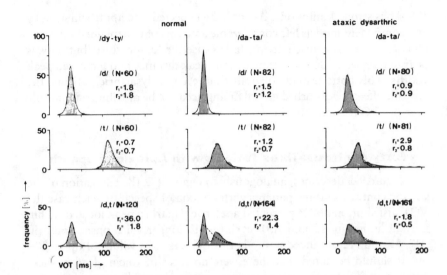

FIGURE 9-2. VOT distributions of initial /d/ (top panels), /t/ (middle panels), and /d,t/ (bottom panels) in a normal subject before /y/ (left column) and /a/ (middle column), and in a patient with ataxic dysarthria before /a/ (right column). *Broken lines:* one-component fitting; *Solid lines:* two-component fitting. In cases where two identical or nearly identical models resulted, they could not be separated graphically. In the left bottom panel, the one-component model yielded a precise fit of the /d/-peak and was zero over the rest of the VOT domain.

over a broader VOT range than its voiced counterpart. In the normal subject, the peak locations of /dy/ and /ty/ (A) were shifted upwards, although not uniformly, in relation to /da/ and /ta/ (B). This conformed to expectations, since for aerodynamical reasons the onset of voicing relates to the rate of vocal tract opening during release (Klatt, 1973). The dysarthric patient's /d/- and /t/-peaks were located 10 and 5 ms higher than the corresponding values of the normal subject and he presented a considerable number of outliers in his productions of /t/. These tokens deserve some consideration: since they deviate away from the category boundary they are not susceptible of being phonemic errors and therefore give account of the potential motor aberrations in this patient. Regarding the few /d/-tokens with abnormally high VOT values, this would mean that a motor explanation is also applicable, although a template-matching procedure would categorize these deviations as phonemic errors.

In the lumped distributions, clear bimodal patterns resulted for the normal subject. There was a considerably larger interval between the two peaks in the /dy/-/ty/-pairs as compared to the /da/-/ta/-samples, indicating that the application of fixed intermodal distances (as in Tuller,

1984) has strong limitations. As could be expected, the approximation by one-component models left considerable amounts of unexplained variance. Not so in the dysarthric patient: In his case the lumped distribution was near to unimodal, due to a reduced interpeak distance and increased peak widths. This pattern made obvious that, even in dysarthric patients, the acoustic effects of disturbed glottal timing need not be distributed uniformly over the VOT domain.

Fuzzy Contrasts: Three Patients with Apraxia of Speech

Figure 9-3 describes, analogously to Figure 9-2, the realization of the voicing contrast in three patients with apraxia of speech. In each case the VOT distribution of /d/ presented a relatively marked peak located within normal limits (in A2 and A3) or shifted to longer voice onset times (in A1). A1 and A2 produced a number of outliers with values of up to 200 ms. It should be noted that there were no cases of voicing lead in these patients. In exaggeration of the normal pattern, the productions of /t/ scattered more and lacked prominent peaks. One-component models yielded only poor approximations and even two components left some unexplained variance in A2 and A3. In all cases there was more or less of an overlap between the two stop cognates. The lumped distributions of /d/ and /t/ presented in the bottom panels lacked the clear bimodality of the normal

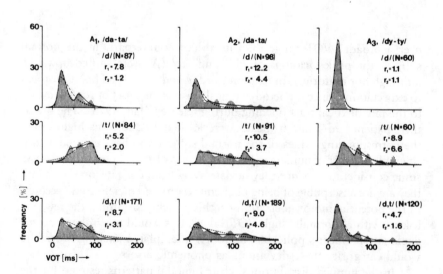

FIGURE 9-3. VOT distributions of initial /d/ (top panels), /t/ (middle panels) and /d,t/ (bottom panels) before /a/ and /y/ in three patients with apraxia of speech. *Broken lines*: one-component fitting; *Solid lines*: two-component fitting.

pattern (Figures 9-1 and 9-2). This was expressed quantitatively by low residual variances obtained in single-component fittings of these distributions.

The question of whether the tokens within the respective overlap regions should be considered as literal paraphasias is addressed in Figure 9-4. This figure depicts the primary component of the /d/-distribution in relation to the /t/-component nearest to /d/ for each of the three speech apraxics of Figure 9-3. Notably, there was no perfect coincidence between these two modes. In all cases, the respective /t/-component was shifted towards higher VOT values and presented a steep slope towards the category boundary. If inappropriate selection of phonetic plans were a salient feature of these patients' speech production deficits it would be difficult to explain why the left tail of the /t/-distributions have virtually returned to zero frequency at the point where the /d/-distributions have their maximum. A similar argument applies to the secondary peak in the /d/-distribution of patient Al (see Figure 9-3). The question of whether this peak should be considered a categorical jump in the /d/-productions involves facing the problem that the /t/ category in this patient had rather fuzzy delimitations with respect to VOT. It is not very reasonable that (phonemic) substitutions of /t/ for /d/ should cluster within a relatively small region whereas the actual attempts at /t/ do not. This argument will appear still more convincing in the light of the results obtained for the nonapraxic aphasics.

One or Two Categories? Another Case of Apraxia of Speech

Figure 9-5 depicts the VOT distributions of initial /d/ and /t/ before /a/ (A) and /y/ (B) of patient A4 as represented by one-component models. The residual variances given in the diagram indicate that these models explained the data well. In contrast to the cases of Figure 9-3 this patient had relatively small peak widths. The VOT measured from her realizations of /daCV/ and /taCV/ raised the question whether a categorical distinction

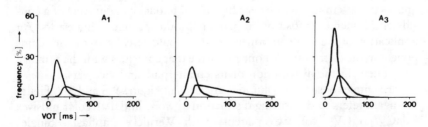

FIGURE 9-4. Primary components of /d/-distributions and lower components of /t/-distributions, isolated from the two-component models of Figure 9-3.

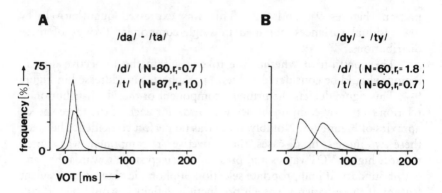

FIGURE 9-5. Overlapping VOT distributions of initial /d/ and /t/ in patient A4 (apraxia of speech) (A) before /a/; (B) before /y/.

between /d/ and /t/ was still available to this patient. The two peaks merged almost completely, with only a slight shift and broadening of the /t/-peak, and the resulting lumped distribution (not plotted) was unimodal. The pattern that emerged from the same patient's realizations of /d/ and /t/ before /y/, however, suggested an affirmative answer to this question. Although there was still a broad overlap between the two categories, two clearly distinct peaks could be observed and there remained no doubt concerning the bimodality of the resulting lumped distribution. Obviously, the altered aerodynamic conditions in the /y/-context helped to unveil the contrast concealed in the VOT distribution of the /da/-/ta/-tokens. Differences in the degree of lingual–laryngeal coupling in the two vowels may also account for the observed effect.

Coupled Modes Two Cases of Wernicke's Aphasia

Assuming that the physical manifestations of a misselected phonetic plan obey the same statistical laws as do the realizations of this plan when appropriately selected, there should be a correspondence between primary and secondary modes in the distributions of phonetic parameters of a considered phoneme opposition in patients producing phonemic errors. An application of the two-component model should reveal a secondary component in the distribution of one phoneme that coincides with the primary component in the distribution of its counterpart and vice versa.

Examples of such distributions are given in Figures 9-6 and 9-7. Figure 9-6 again refers to the voicing distinction in word-initial alveolar plosives (/daCV/–/taCV/) for two patients with Wernicke's aphasia. Single-component fittings in their cases yielded very poor approximations to the empirical VOT distributions of /d/ and /t/, respectively, and a substantial

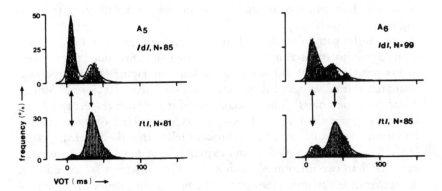

FIGURE 9-6. Cross-coupled models of VOT distributions for /d/ and /t/ in two Wernicke's aphasics.

improvement was achieved by using two-component models. The result was a mutual congruence between primary and secondary modes of /d/ and /t/. For a quantitative assessment of this fact the VOT distribution for each of the two stop cognates was approximated by a two-component model with the requirement that the locations of primary and secondary peaks of the two counterparts coincide (see arrows in Figure 9-6). In the two Wernicke's aphasics such *cross-coupled* models left no more than 1.3% (A5) and 1.9% (A6) of the total variance unexplained. The requirement of coupled components meant no substantial deterioration in the

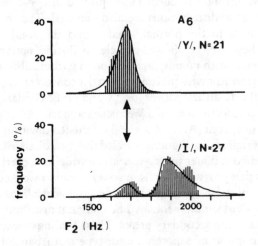

FIGURE 9-7. Cross-coupled models of F2 distributions for /Y/ and /I/ in a patient with Wernick's aphasia.

goodness-of-fit when compared to an independent fitting of the two cognates.

A similar pattern resulted when patient A6 was examined with regard to his capability of discriminating the rounded and unrounded front vowels in his productions of /kɪsən/ and /kysən/. In Figure 9-7 interpolated histograms of F2 values of these vowels are depicted (class width: 50 Hz; 3 interpolation points). The two cognates differed with respect to F2, /y/ assuming generally lower values than its unrounded counterpart /ɪ/. However, a total of 5 out of 27 /ɪ/-tokens fell within the frequency range of /y/. Again, the coupled model explained not much less of the total variance than two uncoupled models did. These patterns suggested that, in the Wernicke's aphasics, the deviant attempts at one member of a minimal pair were tokens of the same type as the majority of attempts at its counterpart. In this respect they contrasted well with the patterns obtained for subjects A1 to A4 (Figures 9-3 to 9-5), in which the requirement of cross-coupling meant a drastic increase in residual variance.

Two-Dimensional Distributions

Like English, German tense vowels differ from their lax counterparts in duration and formant structure (Jørgensen, 1969). This is commonly ascribed to differences in duration and geometrical distinctness of the involved articulatory gesture and to the applied "muscular effort" (Chomsky & Halle, 1968).

Figure 9-8 presents measurements made on the /i:/ – /ɪ/ contrast in the minimal pair /bi:tən/ – /bɪtən/. Vowel durations and the differences of the first two formant frequencies are plotted in two-dimensional scattergrams. Marginal distributions are also depicted. The two examples of Figure 9-8A refer to the normal speaker and the ataxic dysarthric of Figure 9-2. These subjects showed two clearly distinct patterns for the two considered vowels with no misclassification in within-subject discriminant analyses. In agreement with previous reports, a consistent lengthening effect was found in the dysarthric patient (e.g., Gandour & Dardarananda, 1984). Figure 9-8B presents the data of a Wernicke's aphasic (A6) and of a patient with apraxia of speech (A1) In A6, the data clustered within a very limited region. The marginal distributions revealed that two discrete categories were still present in both dimensions, yet with considerable overlap. The point to be made is that gross deviations in vowel duration were correlated with deviations in the formant frequencies, i.e., categorical changes occurred in both dimensions simultaneously. The marginal distributions had cross-coupled primary and secondary peaks. These findings are not compatible with the assumption of a purely motor-type disturbance but are rather indicative of an erroneous selection of phonetic plans.

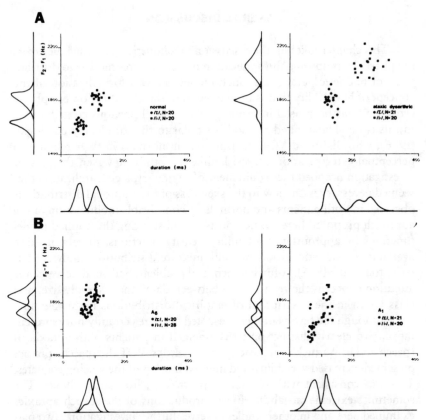

FIGURE 9-8. Scattergrams of durations and formant frequencies for tense and lax vowels. (A) normal subject and ataxic dysarthric; (B) patients with Wernicke's aphasia (A6) and apraxia of speech (A1).

Considering the example of the speech apraxic (Al), his data were centered roughly in the same region as those of the normal subject. His production variability, however, was increased and a broad region of overlap was found in the frequency dimension. In plain contrast to the Wernicke's aphasic, the aberrations in each of the two considered dimensions were dissociated in patient Al. His long vowels presented two marked peaks of almost equal amplitude in their F2–F1 distribution, yet without any corresponding bimodality in the time dimension. Among the short vowels, on the other hand, two instances were found with abnormally high F2–F1 values despite adequately short durations. Such a dissociation cannot be explained by an erroneous selection of phonemic categories, but rather suggests a deficit in realizing either the temporal or the geometric specifications of the required articulatory adjustments in the apraxic speaker.

GENERAL DISCUSSION

This chapter takes up the discussion on phonetic and phonemic errors in aphasia by proposing the application of least squares models to distributions of phonetic parameters. Such models allow a formalization of the concept of bimodality that is fundamental to the classification of aphasic errors and has been used informally in almost all previous contributions to this issue. The applied method is similar to that of Nearey & Hogan (1986), who discussed VOT distributions in normals in their relation to perceptual categorization curves. Unlike this study, however, the present investigation dropped the requirement of symmetry, a genearalization that seemed necessary with view to the skewness of the empirical distributions observed in both patients and normals. A conceivable modification of the approach proposed here would consist in substituting the applied model functions by appropriate probability density functions, thereby making available the statistical tools of finite mixture distribution analysis (Titterington et al., 1985). A further technical problem that still deserves some attention concerns the relationship between data range, sample size, and class width in the description of empirical distributions by histograms.

Although the few examples presented here are certainly not representative, two clearly distinct patterns emerged in patients with apraxia of speech and in Wernicke's aphasics. With regard to VOT the speech apraxics presented increased variability and marked overlap of the voicing cognates. This was consistent with previous reports (e.g., Itoh et al., 1982). The sometimes extreme variability in the productions of the speech apraxics examined here and in other studies deserves further investigation. Two particular sources of variability will be described in a forthcoming article (Ziegler & von Cramon, in press).

In one case, the degree of overlap reached such an extent that a separation of two different categories was no longer possible. This pattern conformed to the results of Freeman and colleagues (1978) or Hoit-Dalgaard and colleagues (1983). However, in a different vowel context, and thus under different aerodynamical conditions, the same patient managed to realize the voicing contrast. This suggested that the patient had not lost the capacity of distinguishing between the phonetic plans corresponding to /d/ and /t/, respectively.

According to the observed VOT patterns, phonemic unity in the productions of voiced and voiceless plosives was preserved in the speech apraxics. The resulting variability in the realizations of single phonemes did not mirror the patient specific realizations of the voicing feature as a whole. This was the crucial difference to the two examined Wernicke's aphasics, who presented clear bimodal patterns with a remarkable congruence in the locations of primary and secondary peaks, operationalized by the concept of cross-coupled components. The results therefore corroborated earlier suggestions according to which aberrations in the sound pattern of Wernicke's aphasics reflect a dysfunction affecting the ✓ discrete structure in the inventory of phonetic plans, whereas patients with apraxia of speech exhibit problems of realizing properly selected phonological units. The results obtained in the analysis of rounded and unrounded vowels were supportive of this syndromal difference. A further and even stronger corroboration was provided by the two-dimensional analysis of the tense–lax contrast in vowels, where a dissociation between the two dimensions in the apraxic speakers provided evidence for deviant realizations of adequate phonological intentions, whereas the Wernicke's aphasics seemed to switch between alternative functional goals. Whether there is a continuum between these two extremes should be subject to closer investigations based on larger patient samples.

The reported data on vowel realizations may be of some interest with respect to the issue raised by Ryalls in Chapter 2. They confirm that segmental aberrations in aphasic speech are not confined to consonants. More comprehensive analyses of both vowel duration and vowel quality can be found in Ryalls (1986). However, bivariate statistics on the tense–lax distinction in aphasics have, to my knowledge, not been presented before.

Most of the results presented here were neither new nor representative. They were rather meant to demonstrate the value of a formalization of existing concepts for promoting discussion on error categories in aphasia. Further applications of least squares fit modeling are suggested, e.g., to spectral cues, to place of articulation, or to the nasal and oral distinction in terms of sound-pressure changes (Ziegler & von Cramon, 1986). Hopefully, this approach can help to analyze the segmental structure of aphasic speech more comprehensively and to increase the validity of our conceptions concerning the nature of aphasic errors.

ACKNOWLEDGMENTS

This study was supported by a BMFT grant. I wish to thank Michael Scherg for making his curve-fitting facilities available to me and for the constant advice he gave after the program was implemented. Detlev von Cramon and Philip Hoole are thanked for their inspiring comments in numerous discussions of data and concepts. I am also indebted to Inge Wiesner for assistance in patient examination and data evaluation.

REFERENCES

Blumstein, S.E. (1981). Phonological aspects of aphasia. In M. T. Sarno (Ed.), *Acquired aphasia*. New York: Academic Press, pp 129–155.

Blumstein, S.E., Cooper, W.E., Zurif, E.B., & Caramazza, A. (1977). The perception and production of voice onset time in aphasia. *Neuropsychologia*, 15, 371–383.

Blumstein, S.E., Cooper, W.E., Goodglass, H., Statlender, S., & Gottlieb, J. (1980). Production deficits in aphasia: A voice-onset time analysis. *Brain and Language*, 9, 153–170.

Bromberger, S. & Halle, M. (1986). On the relationship of phonology and phonetics In J.S. Perkell, & D.H. Klatt (Eds.), *Invariance and variability in speech processes*. Hillsdale, NJ, London. Lawrence Erlbaum Associates, pp 510–520.

Chomsky, Y.N., & Halle, M. (1968). *The sound pattern of english*. New York: Harper & Row.

Fowler, C.A. (1985). Current perspectives on language and speech production: A critical overview. In R.G. Daniloff (Ed.), *Speech science*. London: Taylor & Francis, pp 193–278.

Freeman, F.J., Sands, E.S., & Harris, K.S. (1978). Temporal coordination of phonation and articulation in a case of verbal apraxia: A voice onset time study. *Brain and Language*, 6, 106–111.

Gandour, J., & Dardarananda, R. (1984). Prosodic disturbance in aphasia: Vowel length in Thai. *Brain and Language*, 23, 206–224.

Hewlett, N. (1985). Phonological versus phonetic disorders: Some suggested modifications to the current use of the distinction. *British Journal of Disorders of Communication*, 20, 155–164.

Hoit-Dalgaard, J., Murry, T., & Kopp, H.G. (1983). Voice onset time production and perception in apraxic subjects *Brain & Language*, 20, 329–339.

Huber, W., Poeck, K., Weniger, D., & Willmes, K. (1983). Aachener Aphasie Test (AAT). Göttingen, Toronto, Zürich: Hogrefe.

Itoh, M., Sasanuma, S., Tatsumi, I.F., Murakami, S., Fukusako, Y., & Suzuki, T. (1982). Voice onset time characteristics in apraxia of speech. *Brain & Language*, 17, 193–210.

Jörgensen, H.P. (1969). Die gespannten und ungespannten Vokale in der norddeutschen Hochsprache mit einer spezifischen Untersuchung der Struktur ihrer Formantfrequenzen. *Phonetica*, 19, 217–245.

Klatt, D.H. (1973). Voice onset time, frication and aspiration in word-initial consonant clusters. *Journal of Speech & Hearing Research*, 18, 686–706.

Linnell, P. (1979). *Psychological reality in phonology. A theoretical study*. Cambridge: The University Press.

Lisker, L. & Abramson, A.S. (1964). A cross-language study of voicing in initial stops: Acoustical measurements. *Word*, 20, 384–422.

Nearey, T.M. & Hogan, J.T. (1986). Phonological contrast in experimental phonetics: Relating distributions of production data to perceptual categorization curves. In J.J. Ohala & J.J. Jaeger (Eds.), *Experimental Phonology*. Orlando, FL: Academic Press, pp 141–161.

Ryalls, J.H. (1986). An acoustic study of vowel production in aphasia. *Brain and Language*, 29, 48–67.

Scherg, M., & von Cramon, D. (1985). Two bilateral sources of the late AEP as identified by a spatio-temporal dipole model. *Electroencepholography Clinical Neurophysiology*, 62, 32–44.

Shinn, P., & Blumstein, S.E. (1983). Phonetic disintegration in aphasia: Acoustic analysis of spectral characteristics for place of articulation. *Brain and Language,* 20, 90–114.

Titterington, D.M., Smith, A.F.M., & Makov, U.E. (1985). Statistical analysis of finite mixture distributions. Chichester: John Wiley & Sons.

Tuller, B. (1984). On categorizing aphasic speech errors. *Neuropsychologia,* 22, 547–557.

Ziegler, W. (1984). What can the spectral characteristics of stop consonants tell us about the realization of place of articulation in Broca's aphasia? A reply to Shinn and Blumstein. *Brain and Language,* 23, 167–170.

Zeigler, W., & Hoole, P. (in press). Categorical perception of the voiced-voiceless contrast in aphasic speech. Proceedings of the 11th Congress of Phonetic Sciences. (Tallinn, USSR).

Ziegler, W., and von Cramon, D. (1986). Timing deficits in apraxia of speech. *European Archives Psychiatric and Neurological Sciences,* 236, 44–49.

Ziegler, W. & von Cramon, D. (in press). VOT production in aphasia: Lexical and contextual influences. Proceedings of the 11th Congress of Phonetic Science. (Tallinn, USSR).

Relative Timing of Sentence Repetition in Apraxia of Speech and Conduction Aphasia

R.D. Kent
Malcolm R. McNeil

The relative timing of phrase or sentence production by persons with aphasia or apraxia of speech is difficult to study not only because these disorders are poorly understood but also because relative timing even in normal speech production is a subject of few facts and conflicting theories. Hypotheses about relative timing should be derived from a theory or model of sentence production. Unfortunately, there is no generally accepted, or even reasonably complete, theory or model for this purpose. Several obstacles loom before anyone who would attempt to develop such a theory. One of these obstacles is the difficulty of incorporating into a single theoretical framework the various component processes involved in the production of fluent speech. Included among these processes are utterance formulation (syntactic and semantic planning), phonologic assembly, speech motor control, self-monitoring to verify accuracy and correct errors if necessary, and appropriate integration of cognitive-thematic processing with affective information. Although it is not the central purpose of this chapter to discuss a theoretical framework that embraces these issues, we think that some effort in this direction may promote continuity of thinking. Therefore, the first part of this paper presents theoretical perspectives on the formulation and production of phrases or sentences.

AN INFORMATION-PROCESSING MODEL OF VERBAL FORMULATION AND SPEECH PRODUCTION

One recent model was presented by Bock (1982). Bock's information processing model has been adapted in Figure 10-1. The primary modification is inclusion of an *affective arena*, which takes into consideration

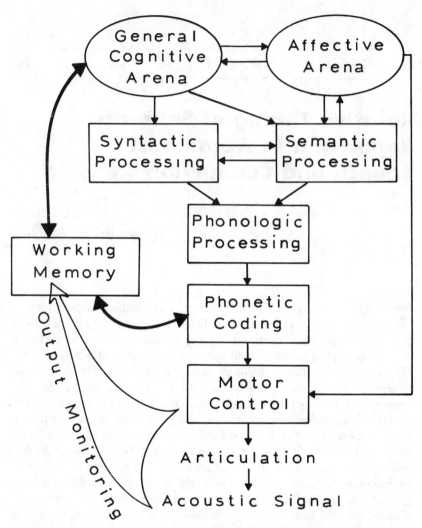

FIGURE 10-1. Major components of an information processing model of sentence formulation and production. The thick lines with double arrows indicate processes that normally require deployment of working memory. Output monitoring is based on information from some or all of the following: motor instructions, articulatory movements, and acoustic signal. (Adapted from Bock, 1982).

affective reactions that contribute to, and accompany verbal formulation and speech production. A brief description of the model is given here. The interested reader should see Bock's paper for a fuller discussion of the issues and supporting data.

Within the *general cognitive arena*, thought is formulated as non-linguistic propositions or relations. It may be regarded as the sphere of conscious awareness and intentional action. This arena includes a referential component that translates or codes the nonlinguistic representation of thought into a format that can be used by the linguistic system. This translation or coding is accomplished by operations called schematization and framing. Schematization organizes nonverbal material into an established pattern that relates the various components of goal-directed events. Such a schema was proposed by Lichtenstein and Brewer (1980) as a "plan" schema. The schema might consist of the specified goal of some actor, together with a sequence of subgoals through which actions are determined to achieve the primary goal. It is possible for schemata to be iterated at different levels, such that subgoals can be schematized within superordinate schemata. Framing (Chafe, 1977) follows schematization when sufficient details are available to formulate a verbal expression suitable to the communicative goals and constraints. Framing is accomplished by the selection of participants and the assignment of participants to roles.

Bock summarizes the *referential arena* as producing a relational structure that "can be neutrally described as a proposition or set of propositions that structure and segment nonlinguistic conceptual patterns." The components and relations that constitute these propositions are processed in the semantic arena.

Bock's model has been modified here to include an *affective arena* that is closely coupled to, but separate from, the *general cognitive arena*. Affective states are determined by cognitive operations, various internal (visceral) states, and by associational mechanisms operating on semantics. The *affective arena* acts directly on motor mechanisms of linguistic expression so that emotional factors may facilitate or interfere with such expressions (see the review in Kent, 1984). Moreover, because the *affective arena* interacts with the *general cognitive arena*, affective reactions can influence cognitive processes.

Syntactic and semantic processing are highly interactive, as indicated by the double arrows between them in Figure 10-1. Semantic processing identifies lexical concepts that match propositions formulated in the *general cognitive arena*. Recent evidence indicates that lexicalization proceeds in two stages, a relatively abstract, prephonological stage and a second stage of phonological realization (Kempen & Huijbers, 1983). Semantic processing in the model of Figure 10-1 can be likened to the L1 (prephonological) stage described by Kempen and Huijbers. The lexical concept thus identified is given a phonological realization in the L2 stage. Thus, lexicalization subtends both semantic and phonological processing.

The two-stage hypothesis may explain certain language abnormalities in the aphasias. First, it is noteworthy that neologistic utterances in jargon aphasia may be preceded by a hesitation pause (Butterworth, 1979). This result detracts somewhat from the common clinical description of these disorders as "fluent" aphasias and illustrates the sensitivity of the output utterance to formulation impairments. Second, O'Connell (1981) reported an analysis of neologistic jargon aphasia in which the neologisms were considered to have a complex origin: (1) correctly retrieved words were subjected to complex, simultaneous paraphasias; (2) incorrectly retrieved words were subjected to further disruption in phonological realization; and (3) recombinations of units from previous utterances were selected to replace target words that either were not retrieved, or were partially or wholly retrieved but could not be correctly specified phonologically because of competition from unsuppressed previously activated elements. The third relationship to aphasia is that effective procedures to facilitate word retrieval vary with the nature of the aphasic person's impairment and it appears that facilitating procedures may be categorized roughly as semantic or phonological (Goodglass, 1983).

Because semantic processing is not concurrently linked to phonological representation, semantic and syntactic processing may interact before phonological decisions are completed. Another consequence is that semantic and syntactic information is available for phonological processing. The mutual regard of semantic and syntactic processing is a feature of much recent work in both linguistics and verbal processing (see Bock, 1982, for discussion of this point). Semantic decisions often carry syntactic privileges and syntactic decisions can in turn influence lexical choices that can be accommodated to the nascent syntax. This interactivity accords with the notion that the first few words of a sentence (typically the noun phrase) are uttered even while the remainder of the utterance is being formulated (Lindsley, 1975, 1976; Bock, 1982; Kempen & Huijbers, 1983). In other words, speakers often begin to produce an utterance before they know completely what they are going to say.

Bock noted that mismatches between syntactic and lexical processing can arise because lexical information is retrieved in parallel but with different time courses for different words. Eventually, both words and syntax must be reconciled to yield serial output, and the need for adjustments between them increases as the discrepancy between the size of the utterance planning unit and the size of the articulatory unit increases. Recent experiments indicate that the former is roughly the size of the clause (Ford & Holmes, 1978; Garrett, 1980) whereas the latter is essentially phrasal (Lindsley, 1975; Gee & Grosjean, 1983).

Information supplied from semantic and syntactic processing is used by the phonological processor, and it is at this stage that the lexical concept becomes phonologically evident as a word. In addition, it is in between the semantic and phonological processing that the "tip of the tongue" phenomenon (Brown & McNeill, 1966) may come about. That is, a lexical concept can be accessed before its phonological form is realized and it is in the search for phonological representation (The L2 stage of Kempen & Huijbers, 1983) that the "tip of the tongue" experience occurs.

It is assumed that in normal fluent adult speech, the syntactic, semantic and phonological processing ordinarily are automatic processes, meaning that thay do not require capacity in working memory. In Figure 10-1, connecting arrows are drawn between working memory and both the *general cognitive arena* and the *phonetic coding* components. However, speakers are flexible in the deployment of automatic and controlled processing. Bock discusses the thesis that language development may be viewed in part as a conversion from controlled to automatic processing for syntactic, semantic, and phonological operations.

The phonological representation is not suitable to govern an acceptable articulatory output. Rather, phonetic coding has to be applied to the phonological representation before motor instructions can be issued (Tatham, 1970; Carney & Severeid, 1974; Nolan, 1983; Rosenbek, Kent, & LaPointe, 1984). After phonetic coding, the utterance, or some fragment of it, is given form as a movement pattern.

Bock had relatively little to say about the phonetic and motor control components of her model, and the representation of these components in Figure 10-1 gives little idea of the complexities and uncertainties that surround phonetic decisions and motor regulation. As Meyer and Gordon (1985) observed, the organization of speech production has been conceptualized in several different ways. Some of the more frequently mentioned alternatives are shown in Figure 10-2, in which candidate representatives are displayed at three levels of organization: (1) a multiunit representation based on networks or sequences; (2) a basic unit of phonetic or prearticulatory representation; and (3) motor control of the speech system.

The topmost level in Figure 10-2 can be conceptualized as conceptual-dependency networks (Schank, 1972), surface-structure sequences of words (Chomsky, 1965), a syntagma, or rhythmic grouping of syllables (Kozhevnikov & Chistovich, 1965; Boomer & Laver, 1968), or an articulatory phrase (Lindsley, 1975; Gee & Grosjean, 1983). Matters are complicated further by the possibility that more than one multiunit representation is involved, e.g., in a hierarchical organization, or in an accommodation between different representations (as may be the case if the utterance planning unit is different from the articulatory unit).

The second level in Figure 10-2 shows several possibilities for the basic unit of speech representation. The syllable, phoneme, allophone, and feature all have been suggested to be the basic unit. Moreover, some or all of these units might be included in a hierarchical organization, e.g., phonetic features might be nested within allophonic decisions, allophones nested within phonemic decisions, and phonemes nested within syllables. Evidence has been presented for each unit in some aspect of speech production. Thus, either all of these units are in fact involved in speech or it must be shown that a parsimonious account of speech organization can be given by just one or a few of them.

The third level in Figure 10-2, that of motor control, also has no dearth of choices. The spatial articulatory target is a kind of a snapshot of the articulatory configuration to be achieved for a particular control unit. For

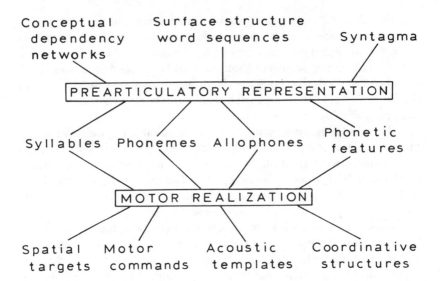

FIGURE 10-2. Levels of organization presumably involved in the articulation of a sentence or other word string. The first level is that of a sequence or network of units that relate to syntactic, lexical and phonological decisions. Candidates at this level are conceptual dependency networks (Schank, 1972), surface-structure sequences of words (Chomsky, 1965), and the syntagma (Kozhevnikov & Chistovich, 1965; Boomer & Laver, 1968). The sequences or networks are converted to smaller units in a prearticulatory representation, which might be based on one or more of the following: syllables (Kozhevnikov & Chistovich, 1965; Liberman, 1970; MacKay, 1972, 1974), phonemes (Fromkin, 1973; Shattuck-Hufnagel & Klatt, 1979), allophones (Wickelgren, 1969; Liberman, 1970; Tatham, 1970), or phonetic features (Jakobson, Fant, & Halle, 1951; Chomsky & Halle, 1968). The units in the prearticulatory representation are thought to have a motor realization as one of the following: spatial articulatory targets (Henke, 1966; MacNeilage, 1970; Mermelstein, 1973), motor commands (Fromkin, 1966; Liberman et al., 1967), acoustic templates (Ladefoged et al., 1972; Lindblom, Lubker, & Gay, 1979), coordinative structures (Fowler et al., 1980; Kelso, Tuller, & Harris, 1980).

example, if the phonetic segment (allophone) is taken to be the control unit, then a spatial articulatory target would be defined for each allophone. The motor command is a presumably invariant neural instruction for each control unit. The strongest proponents of this idea were the investigators from Haskins Laboratories, who also proposed the motor theory of speech perception. Acoustic templates are sound patterns that may be associated with one or more articulatory goals. For example, a goal of lowered formant frequencies for a rounded vowel can be accomplished either by lip protrusion (rounding) or by depression of the larynx. Either of these actions has the result of lengthening the vocal tract and therefore lowering the formant frequencies. A more recent candidate at the level of motor control is the coordinative structure, which may be defined as a group of muscles acting together to produce a particular action such that the degrees of freedom of the group are reduced compared to the total degrees of freedom of the individual muscles. It is assumed that coordinative structures can be modulated by factors such as rate of speech or stress, so that changes in speaking rate or stress can be accounted for by modulation of coordinative structures rather than by a necessity for an entirely different plan of action.

A current controversy in speech motor control that holds profound implications for speech timing is the issue of motor programs. First, is it necessary or desirable to propose that motor programs for speech exist? Second, if the answer to the first question is positive, then what is the structure and content of a speech motor program? Reed (1982) has argued against the concept of programming in motor control generally. However, the idea of a motor program continues to guide much of the thinking about speech production and related motor activities such as typewriting (Sternberg, Monsell, Knoll, & Wright, 1978). The most useful concept of motor program seems not to be the extreme version, in which central commands are generated completely without reliance on feedback. Sternberg and colleagues allow that sequence control can involve both advance planning and feedback, particularly if the latter serves as a cue to trigger onsets of subunits in a sequence or to provide information for an error-control process. Sternberg and colleagues conducted experiments on speech and typewriting to determine the latencies and durations of rapid movement sequences in a reaction-time paradigm. They concluded from their results that sequence control in these tasks could be conceptualized as the following three-stage process: (1) retrieval proceeds as a self-terminating sequence search through a nonshrinking buffer, i.e., the search continues until the unit is found, but the preplanned units remain in the buffer even after they have been found; (2) an unpacking stage separates the constituents of a retrieved unit; and (3) a common stage issues the appropriate sequence of commands to the muscles.

Shaffer (1982) proposed that the reproducible temporal pattern of a motor performance is the result of a schedule in a motor program. The schedule is the means by which the motor system can generate a movement to the next temporal target, using a previous target as a reference point in planning the movement trajectory. Shaffer saw the schedule as affording both the capacity to anticipate targets in space and time and to coordinate movements within the limits of a given schedule. Because Shaffer assumes that the motor control system has a timekeeper role to regulate the time scale of movement trajectories, it is capable of making adjustments for speaking rate, stress, and other prosodic and paralinguistic variables (cf. Rosenbaum et al., 1986). This motor-control system also is thought to be equipped with a scan or look-ahead capability so that it can anticipate movement requirements by inspection of the motor sequence to be performed. This advance planning of the output string might explain several aspects of speech behavior: (1) it is the means for anticipation of movement targets and the determination of supplementary background information such as respiratory requirements for an utterance; (2) the scan allows the grouping of motor commands to form compound movement trajectories; and (3) the look-ahead principle accounts for certain sequencing errors because the scanning operation can confuse context information with order information.

Shaffer's (1982) conception of a motor program is explicit in his comment that: "For a fluent nonrepetitive action to unfold in an orderly temporal pattern of movement, information relevant to the space-time coordinates of the successive movements must be generated ahead of the action so that it is available to the motor system when it is required" (p. 422).

The *affective arena* is shown as having a linkage to motor control in part because emotional state can influence motor activity, e.g., vocal tremor, respiratory unevenness, tensing of the musculature. This linkage also is shown as a reflection of the dissociation between volitionally induced movements and emotionally induced movements. For example, lesions of the cortical strip or corticobulbar projections interfere with voluntary retraction of the mouth but not with bilateral smile. Lesions affecting the extrapyramidal system result in "mimetic facial paralysis" in which voluntary use of the facial muscles is retained but spontaneous emotional movements are not. Kent (1984) has reviewed clinical evidence for the role of emotion in the speech and language behavior of individuals with neurologic disorders. Although the evidence is largely anecdotal, several reports attest to the effects of emotion on verbal responses. The voluntary motor system involves transmission of impulses to the cranial nerve nuclei via the pyramidal tract. Emotional motor responses are transmitted by the phylogentically older extrapyramidal system, which may be thought of as a group of highly interactive neural circuits.

Recent work by Lynch and colleagues, summarized in Lynch (1985), indicates that the physiologic response to speaking is complex and has pronounced cardiovascular implications. Generally, when a person talks, regardless of subject of conversation, the person's blood pressure increases. Observations during cardiac catheterization demonstrated that during quiet talking, increases occurred in cardiac output, central aortic pressure and heart rate. Because blood pressure increases also occur during signing by deaf persons, it appears that the primary factor in producing blood pressure increase is human communication itself and not the motor system that accomplishes communication. Furthermore, blood pressure elevation during speaking appears to be proportionately greater for the elderly than for younger persons. Lynch commented, "These increases were at times so great that we wondered whether some elderly persons might find it particularly difficult to communicate, or become emotionally agitated and quick-tempered with others, or even be susceptible to mental confusion when they talked" (Lynch, 1985, p. 146). One may well wonder if the aphasic individual, who is frequently frustrated with the communication process, exhibits even more serious cardiovascular reactions to speech.

MONITORING

Self-monitoring is an integral part of verbal formulation and speech production. Because of the vulnerability of these processes to error, speakers continually monitor their output to verify that what they have uttered accords with their intentions. When errors are detected, rather systematic correction processes are brought into play (Levelt, 1983). Effective self-monitoring requires that the perceptual processing of self-monitoring is coordinated with production mechanisms. Delayed auditory feedback is one way of interfering with a speaker's self-monitoring.

Monitoring performs two functions (Levelt, 1983). The first is a matching function with two aspects: (1) parsed aspects of inner and outer speech are compared with the speaker's intention to determine if the actual utterance corresponds with the intended expression; and (2) the parsed information for inner and outer speech is compared with production standards to detect speech errors and syntactic flaws as well as to monitor rate, loudness, and other prosodic features. The second monitoring function is to generate instructions for correction or adjustment. Whenever an error or nonstandard production is detected, the monitor must alter the formulator and supply corrective information. When the error is serious, the speaker usually stops and restarts. Levelt observed that, "This restarting is not neutral with respect to the interrupted utterance, it usually reinstalls some of the parsed properties of the original utterance" (p. 50). The supply of context for repair of the error aids the listener in solving a continuation problem—how to relate the speaker's repair to the flawed utterance.

Another type of monitoring was described by Garney and Dell (1984), who reviewed evidence for a prearticulatory editor that monitors the planned output of speech. Semantic information is available to this monitoring operation, thus enabling comparison of lexical decisions with prearticulatory sequences. Presumably, this prearticulatory monitor could be vulnerable to impairment in neurologic disorders of phonologic processing.

The process of self-monitoring is poorly understood in both normal speakers and disordered speakers. However, some writers have proposed that aspects of self-monitoring explain some of the characteristics in aphasia or apraxia of speech. McCarthy and Warrington (1984) concluded from the task specificity of aphasic speech performance that speech production has at least two routes of processing. One of these is of special interest here: a nonsemantic route was thought to serve as (1) a feedback loop in error monitoring and word selection; and (2) a way of refreshing or accessing material in an auditory input buffer. This nonsemantic route, which is principally an auditory–phonetic transcoding process, was hypothesized to be impaired in conduction aphasia. The other processing route involves semantic processing in a circuit that includes verbal comprehension, semantic and phonological transcoding, and the articulatory output system. This route was thought to be damaged in transcortical motor aphasia.

Given the importance of self-monitoring in speech, it is possible that impaired speakers alter their speaking patterns to enable more effective monitoring. One suggestion along this line was offered by Dubois and colleagues (1964, 1973), who suggested that a speaking behavior they described as "syllabification" may come about as the speaker tries to facilitate auditory self-monitoring. Syllabification is a speaking pattern in which words are spoken with halting syllable transitions and equally stressed syllables. Kent and Rosenbek (1983) apparently referred to a similar speaking pattern in their acoustic descriptions of "syllable segregation" and "articulatory prolongation" in apraxia of speech. It would not be surprising if speakers with a phonetic or motoric disorder altered their rate, rhythm and other characteristics of speech to promote the effectiveness of self-monitoring. However, it can be difficult to separate such a deliberate adjustment of the speaking pattern from the unavoidable motoric effects of neural damage.

CONDUCTION APHASIA

Conduction aphasia is thought to impair primarily repetition performance and to have relatively little effect on spontaneous speech and comprehension. In addition, this disorder is associated with frequent phonemic paraphasias on nearly all tests requiring a verbal response. Beyond this surface description of the disorder, there are numerous interpretations of exactly what causes conduction aphasia. Specifically, conduction aphasia has been described as:

1. The consequence of an anatomical disconnection between Wernicke's area, which presumably stores the acoustic representation of words, and Broca's area, which presumably stores the motor representation of words (Geschwind, 1965).
2. A disruption in auditory verbal short-term memory (Warrington, Logue, & Pratt, 1971; Warrington & Shallice, 1972).
3. A general deficit in phonemic coding (Brown, 1975).
4. An impairment of auditory–phonologic transcoding (McCarthy & Warrington, 1984).

5. A deficit in the "first stage of motor encoding" representing a difficulty in maintaining a distinct acoustic image of a target word (Yamadori & Ikumura, 1975).
6. A result of damage at the level of the "first articulation" (Dubois et al., 1964, 1973).
7. A dysfunction in "pre-articulatory programming" in the face of relatively intact speech monitoring and a stable working memory (Kohn, 1984).
8. A deficiency in the generation and maintenance of an abstract phonological code (Friedrick, Glenn, & Marin, 1984).
9. Not a unitary disorder at all (Shallice & Warrington, 1977; Blumstein et al., 1980).

Diverse as these explanations may be, two primary theories about the impairment in conduction aphasia stand out. One is an impairment in phonetic-motor operations and the other is an impairment in the auditory representation available to these operations. Kohn (1984) presented data that she interpreted as meaning that the auditory-phonetic representation in conduction aphasia is not particularly impaired. If her interpretation is correct, then the most likely explanation of this disorder lies in an impairment of phonetic-motor operations. It is unclear if the impairment is primarily in the phonetic representation, the motor component, or both. Nor is it clear why the impairment should occur more for repetition than for spontaneous speech.

APRAXIA OF SPEECH

Apraxia of speech is no less controversial than conduction aphasia. Much of the disagreement over nosology, diagnosis, and theory was reviewed by Rosenbek, Kent, and LaPointe (1984). It appears that the term apraxia of speech (or its variants such as verbal apraxia) is gaining favor in the recent clinical literature, but a review of clinical studies is frustrated by the appearance of many other names that denote an apparently similar, if not the same, disorder. Among these terms are aphemia, anarthria, apraxic dysarthria, motor aphasia, cortical dysarthria, and phonetic disintegration. The early descriptions of apraxia of speech emphasized errors at the phonemic level, especially substitutions but also additions and distortions. Attention also was drawn to the prosody of apraxic speech, typically described as slow, labored, and groping. This speech disorder was considered to result most frequently following infarctions of the middle cerebral artery of the dominant cerebral hemisphere. Apraxia of speech is often, but not always, associated with Broca's aphasia and there is evidence of a clinicoanatomic relationship between them (Seinsch, 1981).

The more recent descriptions of apraxia of speech have indicated that the speech abnormalities go far beyond the phonemic substitutions that dominated the early clinical impressions (for a review, see Rosenbek, Kent, & LaPointe, 1984). In particular, acoustic and physiologic studies have shown that apraxic speech is associated with several types of coordination or timing errors. Weismer and Fennell (1985) reported that neurologically impaired speakers, including two with "apraxic-sounding speech" had stable relative timing in sentence production across changes in speaking rate, despite abnormalities in segment, word, and phrase durations. The identification of these error patterns has strengthened the argument that apraxia of speech is at least partly a result of disrupted motor control processes. Many writers describe apraxia of speech as a "motor programming disorder."

Lesser (1978) summarized much of the literature on apraxia of speech by describing three levels of organization and explanation of the disorder. The first, the *neuromuscular approach*, accounts for articulatory and prosodic abnormalities by positing a breakdown in the neuromuscular organization that controls the initiation and sequencing of speech sounds. The second, the *phonological encoding approach*, interprets phonological errors as encoding disturbances that follow lawful linguistic patterns. The third, the *central phonological approach*, conceptualizes the disorder as a disruption in central phonological organization reflected in both speech and comprehension.

APRAXIA OF SPEECH VIS-A-VIS CONDUCTION APHASIA

At one level, apraxia of speech and conduction aphasia are distinct disorders of communication. Apraxia of speech affects both spontaneous and repeated utterances and usually is associated with (and sometimes even classified as) nonfluent aphasia. Conduction aphasia is associated with an impairment of repetition that contrasts with less impaired spontaneous speech. Conduction aphasia therefore is usually classified as a fluent aphasia. However, at the level of explanation, apraxia of speech and conduction aphasia would seem to involve similar mechanisms. Both have been interpreted as resulting from damage to phonologic or motor systems of speech production. It becomes of special interest, then, to compare the repetition responses of persons with these two types of speech disorder.

Interpretation of the deficit or damage in apraxia of speech and conduction aphasia is hindered by the lack of a generally accepted model of speech production. Although writers of clinical articles frequently allude to various processes or levels of phonologic assembly, phonologic retrieval, prearticulatory or articulatory motor programming, and motor execution, in fact such processes or levels are poorly defined. We have tried to point out the inadequacies of current understanding in the preceding review. Despite the admitted shortcomings in conceptualizations of verbal formulation and speech production, we think it important to consolidate facts and interpretations in a comprehensive model, and it is for this reason that we have discussed a modified version of Bock's information processing model of sentence production. We think that this model is a useful theoretical framework for the understanding of the various processes that may be impaired in aphasia and kindred disorders.

Figure 10-3 is a summary of recent conceptions of speech processing performed by various regions of the cortex. This illustration is based on discussions in Darley, Aronson, and Brown (1975), Mlcoch and Noll (1980), and McCarthy and Warrington (1984). The model is relevant to both the verbal repetition task and the suspected disruption of speech processing in apraxia of speech and conduction aphasia. Anatomic localization is shown for the five components of speech and language processing based on suggestions by Darley and colleagues and Mlcoch and Noll. However, it should be noted that the localization scheme does not entirely accord with clinicoanatomic reports for apraxia of speech (Rosenbek, Kent, &

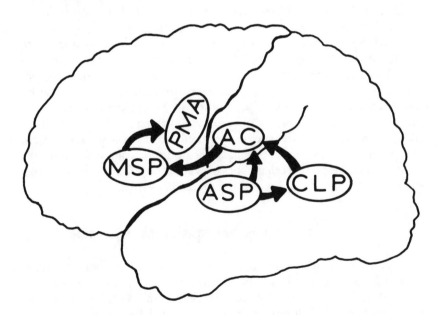

FIGURE 10-3. Diagram of functional components in a model of speech production (based on Darley, Aronson, & Brown, 1975; Mlcoch & Noll, 1980). ASP = auditory speech processor; CLP = central language processor; AC = articulatory coder; MSP = motor speech programmer, PMA = primary motor area.

LaPointe, 1984) or conduction aphasia (Damasio & Damasio, 1980). The auditory speech processor (ASP) is responsible for phonetic perception of auditory signals and for the selection of phonemes in speech production. The anatomic location of the ASP is in the midtemporal lobe region of the dominant hemisphere. Mlcoch and Noll refer to the output of the ASP as the "phonological configuration of the intended utterance," but it seems to us that the output would be more correctly described as a phonetic representation, particularly for the processing of a heard speech signal.

The ASP forwards phonetic information to the central language processor (CLP) or to the articulatory coder (AC). The CLP located in the angular gyrus region accomplishes a semantic interpretation of the phonetic information and encodes the semantic interpretation into a form that is suitable to be passed on to the motor areas. The AC, at the supramarginal-postcentral gyrus region, converts phonetic information into articulatory specifications. Mlcoch and Noll (1980) note that the AC is located at the lesion site for conduction aphasia, but those favoring a disconnection explanation are more likely to identify the lesion in conduction aphasia at the arcuate fasciculus. The alternative routes from the ASP to the CLP or the AC may correspond with McCarthy and Warrington's (1984) proposal for a two-route model of speech production, one being semantic and the other nonsemantic.

Articulatory specifications formulated in the AC are transmitted to the motor speech programmer (MSP), located at the inferior portion of the third frontal convolution. As its name suggests, this component is considered to plan or program the motor response based on the articulatory specifications from the AC. The location of MSP often is taken as the primary lesion site in apraxia of speech. According to Mlcoch and Noll (1980), damage to this area presumably results in errors of incoordination, sequencing, and anticipation. Finally, neuromotor commands from the MSP are issued to the speech muscles by way of the primary motor (PMA), located at the oral-facial area of the precentral gyrus.

MEASURES OF TEMPORAL STRUCTURE IN SPEECH

Several approaches can be taken to describe the temporal structure of speech. One approach is to determine statistics for segment durations (Crystal & House, 1982; Carlson & Granstrom, 1986). Carlson and Granstrom reviewed durational rules formulated from real-speech data bases. Crystal and House determined segment durations for script readings by 14 talkers. The duration density distributions were fit by the two-parameter gamma distribution in which parameter λ indicates the rate of decay of the tail of the distribution and parameter r reflects the displacement of the mode along the time scale. For example, long vowels were associated with a large r-value (5.4) and a small λ-value (0.042), whereas voiced fricatives had a small r-value (4.8) and a large λ-value (0.095). Because the tail of the duration density distribution normally falls less steeply for long vowels than for voiced fricatives, it is likely that listeners may be less tolerant of prolongations of the former than the latter. Pauses also are part of the temporal structure of speech, and listener tolerance of pause durations is expected to vary depending on location of the pause. The shortest pauses normally occur between function words and the words with which they are phonologically connected (Gee & Grosjean, 1983). It appears from the data of Crystal and House (1982) on segments and the data of Gee and Grosjean (1983) on pauses that durations for both of these categories can be predicted as successfully on total duration measures as any other basis. That is, total duration of utterance and total pause time within the utterance provide the basic contextual information within which temporal features can be evaluated.

From most accounts of speech production, one could easily conclude that speaking rate is a fairly constant attribute of an utterance. This impression is reinforced by numerous reports that give a single value of speaking rate. A very different conclusion was drawn by Miller, Grosjean, and Lomanto (1984). They reported that the variation in average syllable duration during conversational speech is quite large—on the order of hundreds of milliseconds. Miller and colleagues analyses indicated that speaking-rate changes in conversation result in large part from changes in articulation rate and not just from variations in pausing. This interpretation casts a different light on rate control from that which is explicit or implicit in most models of speech production. It does not appear that a speaker governs speaking rate by a kind of preset, invariant specification. Rather, rate appears to be, shall we say, dynamic. Indeed, the interesting possibility emerges that speaking with a carefully controlled uniform rate would sound unnatural or perhaps even unpleasant in the long run.

In the remainder of this chapter, we report data on sentence repetition by 3 groups of adult male speakers: normal controls, persons with apraxia of speech, and persons with conduction aphasia. Data are presented for two sentences produced five times each at two speaking rates: control and fast. Acoustic data were obtained on various aspects of the temporal structure of the repeated sentences.

METHODS AND PROCEDURES

Subjects

Eight adult right-handed males served as subjects for this investigation. All were native speakers of English and had speech discrimination of 70% or better at 40 dB HL in at least one ear. Three of these were normal controls, between the ages of 57 and 69 years with an average age of 63 years, 4 months. All control subjects were without a history or evidence of speech, language, cognitive or neurologic deficits as determined by a neurologic examination conducted by a Board Certified Neurologist and by a large battery of standardized speech, language and cognitive tests administered by a certified speech-language pathologist. The most salient of these tests for the purpose of this particular investigation are summarized in Table 10-1. These tests included the Raven Coloured Progressive Matrices (RCPM) (Raven, 1962), the Word Fluency Measure (WFM) (Borkowski, Benton, & Spreen, 1967), the Revised Token Test (RTT) (McNeil & Prescott, 1978), the Porch Index of Communicative Ability (PICA) (Porch, 1967), portions of the Boston Diagnostic Aphasia Examination (BDAE) (Goodglass & Kaplan, 1983), the oral and limb sections of the Apraxia Battery for Adults (ABA) (Dabul, 1979), and a structural-functional speech system evaluation (S-F) (Veterans Administration Hospital Examination, Madison, Wisconsin).

The 3 apraxic subjects ranged in age from 52 to 73, with a mean age of 62 years. They ranged in time post onset from 3 years and 3 months to 5 years and 4 months, with an average of 4 years and 3 months. All subjects were diagnosed as having apraxia of speech (AOS) without concomitant dysarthria and without aphasia to a degree that would interfere with the accomplishment of the task or to a degree that was detectable with the battery of tests administered. Darley's (1982) definition was used for the conceptual determination of aphasia.

The presence of AOS was judged perceptually by two certified speech-language pathologists experienced in the detection of AOS and its differential diagnosis from aphasia and dysarthria. These judgments included the presence of effortful trial-and-error groping on the initiation of speech gestures; frequent single feature sound substitutions; articulation and prosody judged at least as accurate on imitation as on spontaneous speech production on the "cookie theft picture" description from the BDAE; variability of articulation and prosody on repeated trials of the same utterance; articulatory agility, phrase length and melodic line ratings on the BDAE between 1 and 4; and without evidence of weakness or incoordination of the speech musculature upon examination (clinical neurological exam or the S-F exam); or when used for automatic vegetative acts such as chewing, swallowing, and sucking. Other criteria for inclusion in this category was a score at or above the 95th percentile for normal subjects on the average of subtests II, III, V, VI, VII, VIII, X, and XI of the PICA, and a score of 22 or above on the RCPM. The biographical and descriptive data for all subjects are summarized in Table 10-1.

The 2 conduction aphasic subjects were 60 and 62 years of age. Both subjects had a minimum speech discrimination of 70% at 40 dB HL in one ear. They achieved a total score of 103 or above on the average of the

TABLE 10-1. Summary of Biographical and Descriptive Characteristics for Three Normal Control, Three Speech Apraxic and Two Conduction Aphasic Subjects.

Biographic and descriptive measure	N1	N2	N3	A1	A2	A3	C1	C2
Gender	M	M	M	M	M	M	M	M
Age	57	64	69	62	54	72	60	62
S-F Exam.	WNL	WNL	WNL	WNL	WNL	WNL1	WNL2	WNL2
Total RCPM	33	29	31	28	30	28	32	27
Total WFM	30	34	34	4	11	31	16	12
Overall PICA	14.84	14.51	14.53	14.33	14.53	14.96	14.13	14.87
Overall RTT	14.83	14.15	14.88	12.08	12.23	14.07	13.04	13.94
BDAE total aud. comp.	119	117	117	113	118	116	103	114
BDAE Speech ratings:								
Articulatory agility	7	7	7	4	3	1	5	5
Phrase length	7	7	7	4	4	4	5	5
Melodic line	7	7	7	4	4	2	7	5
BDAE sent. rep. total sentences w/o errors	8	8	8	7	1	1	1	3
Apraxia bat. For adults:								
Total Limb	50	50	49	50	48	45	50	50
Total Oral	50	50	49	37	49	43	49	49

WNL = Within Normal Limits; WNL1 = There was a questionable right-sided lingual weakness on clinical examination for this subject; WNL2 = There was a question of oral sensory diminution on clinical examination in this subject.

The subjects used in this study have been used in a series of investigations. In order to maintain coherence across studies, the following subject codes have been used (the subject number used in this study appears first and the master subject code appears second): N1 = N2; N2 = N4; N3 = N5; A1 = A2; A2 = A3; A3 = A4; C1 = C3; C2 = C4.

BDAE auditory comprehension subtests, and at or above the 35th percentile on the PICA overall score. They described the "cookie theft picture" from the BDAE and achieved ratings between 4 and 7 on articulatory agility, phrase length, and melodic line. They were without evidence of effortful trial and error groping on the initiations of speech gestures or frequent single feature sound substitutions. They also presented without evidence of (dysarthria) weakness or incoordination of the speech musculature when used for reflexive-automatic acts such as chewing, swallowing, and sucking as elicited from the ABA, the S-F Examination, or the clinical muscle strength or reflex testing on neurological examination. Subjects demonstrated the presence of literal paraphasias in spontaneous speech or in repetition tasks from the BDAE (literal paraphasia was defined as "the perception of a sound substitution, anticipation, or transposition"). In addition to these descriptive measures, the total of 8 sentences presented to each subject from the BDAE that were repeated without errors, are presented in Table 10-1. Two of the three apraxic and both aphasic subjects had considerable difficulty on this task. Only apraxic subject A1 had a limb or oral nonspeech apraxia as determined by performance on the ABA.

Procedures

The data for this investigation were collected in the context of a larger study designed to evaluate the relationships among EMG, aerodynamic, acoustic, and kinematic measures within and among several subject groups, on multiple experimental tasks chosen for their potential influence on the speech of persons with ataxic dysarthria, conduction aphasia, or apraxia of speech. During the collection of the acoustic data reported here, the subjects were seated approximately 12 inches from a microphone, in a comfortable dental chair, with a set of movement transducers attached to a head-held mount, and affixed to the upper lip, lower lip, and jaw. Each subject also had 6 intramuscular hooked wire electrodes attached to the upper lip, lower lip, and jaw. An oral pressure transducer was also placed in the corner of the mouth throughout the speech tasks. All data were recorded on a 12-channel, FM tape recorder for later digitization and analysis. In addition, all speech was simultaneously recorded on a cassette tape recorder using a high quality condensor microphone, for later perceptual and acoustic analyses.

In this experiment, the subjects were instructed to repeat 15 different words and phrases after each stimulus delivered at a single rate, from a tape recorder. Each stimulus was randomly presented, 5 times, among the other 14 stimuli. Each of 9 different repetition tasks were achieved through subject instructions. These tasks were: *control, fast and slow rate, contrastive stress, gestural reorganization, visual* (reading), *visual plus auditory, multiple repetition*, and *intoning*. Only data from the first 2 tasks, the *control* and *fast rate*, will be reported in this chapter.

During the *control* task, the subjects were instructed to repeat each utterance as closely as possible to the model (segmentally and suprasegmentally). During the fast rate condition, the subjects were instructed to repeat each utterance delivered from the tape recorder except that they were to produce it as fast as possible with as few speech errors as possible. The subjects were continually encouraged to maximize their rate. From the multiple utterances produced under each of these conditions, two stimuli were selected for analysis (utterance #1, *Buy Bobby a poppy*, and utterance #2, *Build a big building*) because they (1) require production of a syllable sequence; (2) are not especially complex phonetically; and (3) lend themselves to a relatively straightforward acoustic segmentation.

From each of these utterances, a sonagram was made using a Kay Digital Spectrograph (Model 7800). From these sonagrams, each of the utterances were segmented into pseudosyllables. The pseudosyllable release and stop were marked as shown in Figure 10-4 using conventional segmentation criteria for stop bursts and vowel segments. Figure 10-4 shows the segmentation based on release (r) and stop (s) features of each pseudosyllable.

From these segmented utterances, measures were made in millimeters and converted to milliseconds for each of the segments (pseudosyllables) (lr-ls, 2r-2s, 3r-3s, 4r-4s, 5r-5s) and the intersegmental durations (ls-2r, 2s-3r, 3s-4r, 4s-5r). From these measures, total and average durations were computed for each trial of the two sentences and for the average of each of the two sentences at each rate condition. In addition, the ratio and percent of the intersegment to segment duration was computed for each trial and for the average of each of the two utterances at each rate condition. These averages are summarized in Tables 10-2, 10-3, 10-4, and 10-5 for the two stimulus utterances produced at the control and fast rate.

A finer segmentation of the word *poppy* from utterance #1 was performed as an analysis of acoustic-phonetic structure. The 5 divisions are illustrated in Figure 10-4. Finally, the F2 (second formant) trajectory was traced for pseudosyllable #4 in utterance #2 to provide an index of the formant structure of a syllable nucleus. Figure 10-4 illustrates the F2 trajectory tracing.

RESULTS

The major focus of the analysis of the sentence repetitions was on the measured durations of the pseudosyllable segments (which we will call simply segment durations in this discussion) and the intersegments (the intervals between succcessive segments). This analysis is illustrated for the

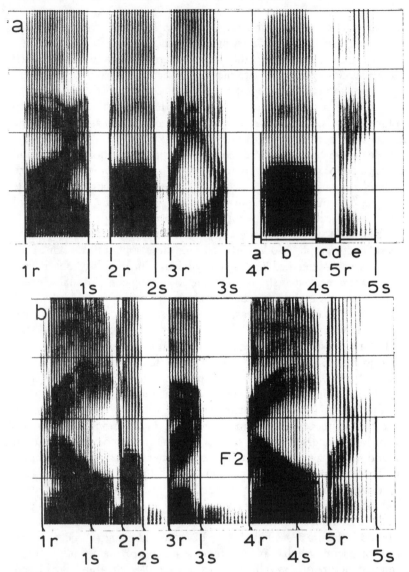

FIGURE 10-4. Spectrograms showing segmentation for duration measurements for the two sentences: *Buy Bobby a poppy* (a) and *Build a big building* (b). Each sentence was segmented into five pseudosyllables defined by an acoustic release (r) and an acoustic closure or stop (s). In addition, an acoustic-phonetic segmentation was made of the word *poppy* to define five phonetic segments a, b, c, d and e, and the F2 trajectory was determined for the first pseudosyllable in *building* (pseudosyllable 4 in spectrogram b).

TABLE 10-2. Mean, Range, and Mean Range of Segment and Intersegment Durations; Mean, Range, and Mean Range of the Percentage of Total Utterance Duration for Segments and Intersegments; Ratio of Intersegment-to-Segment Duration; Percentage of Segment and Intersegment Change from Control-to-Fast Rates for Sentence Repetition #1 *Buy Bobby a poppy* for the Control Rate.

Measurement variable	Subject							
	N1	N2	N3	A1	A2	A3	C1	C2
Number of sentences used in analysis	5	5	5	5	5	4	1	5
M. seg. dur. (ms)	877	824	697	800	1113	1684	1199	1054
R. seg. dur. (ms) (Total R.)	833–949 (116)	766–880 (114)	674–748 (74)	686–870 (184)	1043–1204 (161)	1528–1909 (381)	—	1026–1113 (87)
Seg. M. % utt. dur.	73	79	71	62	65	52	70	78
Seg. R. % utt. dur. (Total R. %)	70–76 (6)	74–82 (8)	69–75 (6)	48–72 (24)	52–71 (19)	46–62 (16)	—	75–80 (5)
M. interseg. dur. (ms)	312	222	281	494	600	1522	685	289
R. interseg. dur. (ms) (Total R.)	263–381 (118)	190–262 (72)	223–307 (80)	318–902 (584)	428–947 (519)	1095–1839 (744)	—	267–348 (81)
Interseg. m. % utt. dur.	27	21	29	38	35	48	43	22
Interseg. R. % utt. dur. (Total R. %)	24–30 (6)	18–26 (8)	25–31 (6)	28–52 (24)	29–48 (19)	38–54 (16)	—	20–25 (5)
Interseg./seg. ratio	0.37	0.27	0.40	0.62	0.54	0.90	0.57	0.27
R. interseg./seg. ratio (Total R.)	0.42–0.32 (0.10)	0.23–0.40 (0.17)	0.33–0.46 (0.13)	0.39–1.08 (0.69)	0.41–0.90 (0.49)	0.62–1.19 (0.57)	—	0.24–0.34 (0.10)
% Seg. control/F.R.	42<	37<	28<	3>	8<	3<	24<	16<
% Interseg. control/F.R.	25<	69<	30<	13<	1>	25<	37<	11<

normal control subjects in Figure 10-5, which shows the pseudosyllable segments in sentence #2 (*Build a big building*) produced at the control and fast rates. The fourth intersegment duration for N3's production is somewhat shorter than the durations for the other normal speakers because a different segmentation criterion had to be used for the fourth pseudosyllable (specifically, the onset of closure for [d]). Also for N3, the results are shown for only three tokens at the fast rate because of irregularities in two of the tokens, which were excluded from analysis. These temporal profiles illustrate the relative stability of the segment and intersegment durations when they are aligned with respect to the release of the initial [b] in the first word of the sentence. In the following two sections,

TABLE 10-3. Mean, Range, and Mean Range of Segment and Intersegment Durations; Mean, Range, and Mean Range of the Percentage of Total Utterance Duration for Segments and Intersegments; Ratio of Intersegment-to-Segment Duration, for Sentence #1 *Buy Bobby a poppy* for the Fast Rate.

Measurement variable	Subject							
	N1	N2	N3	A1	A2	A3	C1	C2
Number of sentences used in analysis	3	3	4	5	5	1	1	5
M. seg. dur. (ms)	627	632	486	843	949	1602	736	765
R. seg. dur. (ms) (Total R.)	608–645 (37)	586–684 (98)	401–543 (142)	735–986 (151)	784–1045 (261)	—	—	690–814 (124)
Seg. M. % utt. dur.	77	76	72	69	61	64	70	77
Seg. R. % utt. dur. (Total R. %)	73–79 (6)	71–81 (10)	64–80 (24)	62–75 (13)	46–69 (23)	—	—	75–79 (41)
M. interseg. dur. (ms)	573	204	153	384	610	917	316	232
R. interseg. dur. (ms) (Total R.)	170–230 (60)	260–242 (82)	137–218 (81)	312–592 (280)	446–914 (468)	—	—	215–244 (29)
Interseg. m. % utt. dur.	23	24	28	31	39	36	30	23
Interseg. R. % utt. dur. (Total R. %)	21–27 (6)	19–29 (10)	20–34 (24)	25–38 (13)	31–54 (23)	—	—	21–25 (4)
Interseg./seg. ratio	0.31	0.32	0.39	0.46	0.64	0.57	0.43	0.30
R. interseg./seg. ratio (Total R.)	0.26–0.37 (0.11)	0.23–0.41 (0.18)	0.25–0.57 (0.32)	0.34–0.60 (0.26)	0.44–1.17 (0.73)	—	—	0.26–0.34 (0.08)

the segment and intersegment durations will be reported for all subjects for whom the requisite data could be determined. Productions excluded from analysis included those with major deviations in syllable sequence (e.g., repetition of a syllable or intrusion of a syllable) and unusually long interruptions in the sentence pattern.

Segment Durations

The average segment durations for both the control and fast rate conditions were considerably longer for both the apraxic and conduction aphasic subjects than for the normal subjects. The only exception among the pathological subjects was A1, whose average segment durations fell within the average normal duration at the control rate but not at the fast rate. While the segment durations summarized in Table 10-2 were greater for C2 than for the normal subjects, the total range of durations (87 ms)

TABLE 10-4. Mean, Range, and Mean Range of Segment and Intersegment Durations; Mean, Range, and Mean Range of the Percentage of Total Utterance Duration for Segments and Intersegments; Ratio of Intersegment-to-Segment Duration; Percentage of Segment and Intersegment Change from Control-to-Fast Rates for Sentence #2 *Build a big building* for the Control Rate.

Measurement variable	Subject							
	N1	N2	N3	A1	A2	A3	C1	C2
Number of sentences used in analysis	5	5	5	5	5	5	—	5
M. seg. dur. (ms)	615	628	542	588	1069	1654	—	706
R. seg. dur. (ms) (M.R.)	557–656 (99)	610–642 (32)	494–583 (89)	531–656 (125)	728–1260 (532)	1449–1832 (383)	—	658–754 (96)
Seg. M. % utt. dur.	60	62	59	58	50	54	—	58
Seg. R. % utt. dur. (M.R. %)	59–61 (2)	60–64 (4)	56–63 (7)	55–64 (9)	41–56 (15)	46–59 (13)	—	56–68 (12)
M. interseg. dur. (ms)	406	387	374	427	1081	1391	—	399
R. interseg. dur. (ms) (M.R.)	377–446 (69)	346–420 (74)	348–420 (72)	369–457 (88)	921–1211 (290)	1129–1805 (676)	—	345–450 (105)
Interseg. M. % utt. dur.	40	38	41	42	50	46	—	42
Interseg. R. % utt. dur. (M.R. %)	39–41 (2)	36–40 (4)	37–44 (7)	36–45 (9)	44–59 (15)	41–54 (13)	—	32–44 (12)
Interseg./seg. ratio	0.66	0.62	0.69	0.73	1.01	0.84	—	0.57
R. interseg./seg. ratio (Total R.)	0.63–0.79 (0.13)	0.57–0.71 (0.14)	0.60–0.79 (0.19)	0.56–0.82 (0.26)	0.77–1.47 (0.70)	0.68–1.16 (0.48)	—	0.37–0.68 (0.31)
% Seg. control/F.R.	19<	17<	34<	1<	21<	14<	—	22<
% Interseg. control/F.R.	40<	10<	48<	13>	1<	44<	—	26<

was within the ranges for the normal subjects for both utterances at both speaking rates. In marked contrast, the ranges for the apraxic subjects greatly exceeded those of the normal and aphasic subjects. For example, for sentence #1 in Table 10-2, the ranges for A1, A2, and A3 were 184, 161, and 381 ms, respectively, whereas the largest range for any of the other subjects was 116 ms (for N1). With only a few exceptions, this general pattern held for both sentences at both rates.

Put in another way, the average percentage of the utterance contributed by the segment durations was consistently smaller for the apraxic subjects in sentence #1, control rate (52–62% in Table 10-2), and tended to be smaller for these subjects in sentence #2, control rate (50–58% in Table 10-4). The average percentage of the utterance contributed by the

TABLE 10-5. Mean, Range, and Mean Range of Segment and Intersegment Durations; Mean, Range, and Mean Range of the Percentage of Total Utterance Duration for Segments and Intersegments; Ratio of Intersegment-to-Segment Duration, for Sentence #2 *Build a big building* for the Fast Rate.

Measurement variable	Subject							
	N1	N2	N3	A1	A2	A3	C1	C2
Number of sentences used in analysis	5	5	3	5	5	1	—	4
M. seg. dur. (ms)	416	431	442	577	700	1260	—	566
R. seg. dur. (ms) (Total R.)	380–446 (66)	374–475 (101)	433–449 (16)	461–650 (189)	586–821 (235)	—	—	416–702 (286)
Seg. M. % utt. dur.	60	58	67	51	40	70	—	66
Seg. R. % utt. dur. (Total R. %)	58–65 (7)	53–60 (7)	66–67 (1)	29–67 (38)	31–46 (15)	—	—	50–74 (24)
M. interseg. dur. (ms)	274	316	219	556	1062	538	—	291
R. interseg. dur. (ms) (Total R.)	239–316 (77)	302–333 (31)	216–221 (5)	302–1108 (806)	839–1639 (800)	—	—	219–409 (190)
Interseg. M. % utt. dur.	40	42	33	49	60	30	—	34
Interseg. R. % utt. dur. (Total R. %)	35–42 (7)	40–47 (7)	33–34 (1)	33–71 (38)	54–69 (15)	—	—	26–50 (24)
Interseg./seg. ratio	0.66	0.73	0.50	0.96	1.52	0.43	—	0.51
R. interseg./seg. ratio (Total R.)	0.54–0.73 (0.19)	0.67–0.87 (0.20)	0.48–0.51 (0.03)	0.50–2.40 (1.90)	1.18–2.23 (1.05)	—	—	0.35–0.98 (0.63)

segment durations was comparable for the normal subjects and for the conduction aphasics.

The increased variability of the apraxic subjects is apparent in the ranges of the percentages and in the total range of the percentages for the segment durations. The apraxic subjects' total ranges for sentence #1 for the control rate (Table 10-2) were from 16 to 24%, while the normal and aphasic subjects ranged from 5 to 8%. Similar differences between the subject group occurred for the other sentences as well. This means that the percentage of the total utterance duration accounted for by the utterance to utterance segment measurements was much more variable for the apraxic subjects than those same utterance segments (pseudosyllables) for the other two subject populations.

In general, the aphasic subjects had average segment durations and ranges that were comparable to the apraxic subjects in the fast rate conditions. This is in opposition to the average durations and variabilities more

Control

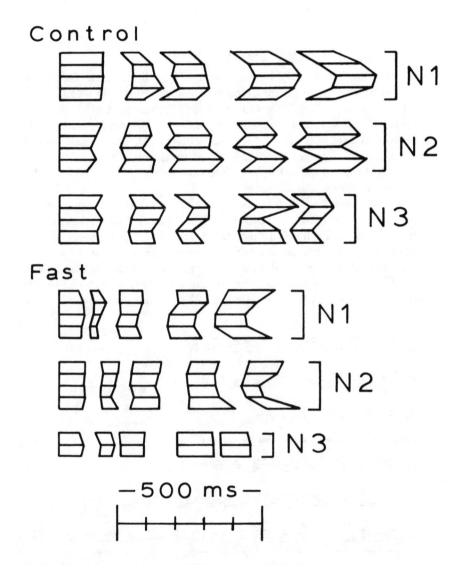

FIGURE 10-5. Temporal profiles for the pseudosyllables in *Build a big building* produced by the three normal talkers five times each at each of the two speaking rates. Durations for each pseudosyllable are joined by lines to form "pseudosyllable islands."

comparable to the normal subjects in the control utterances (e.g., the 24% total segmental range for the fast rate for sentence #2 compared to the 1 and 7% total range for the normal subjects) (Table 10-5).

Intersegment Durations

Utterances produced by the three apraxic subjects at the control rate had substantively longer mean intersegment durations (494–1522 ms for sentence #1 and 427–1391 ms for sentence #2) than those produced by the normal (222–312 ms for sentence #1 and 374–406 ms for sentence #2) and aphasic subjects (289–685 ms for sentence #1). The apraxic subjects' extended intersegment durations ranged from nearly twice to five times as long as the normal and aphasic intersegments (see Tables 10-2 and 10-5 and Figures 10-6 and 10-7).

During the fast rate condition, the aphasic subjects produced average intersegment durations (232–316) within the ranges of the normal subjects (153–573). Figure 10-8 illustrates the results for C2. It should be noted, however, that N1 had considerably longer average intersegment durations than the other normal subjects and longer than he did in that sentence produced at the control rate. The apraxic subjects ranged from 384–1062 ms for the fast rate condition. However, A1 produced a considerably shorter

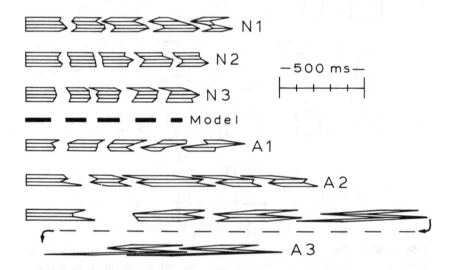

FIGURE 10-6. Temporal profiles for the pseudosyllables in *Buy Bobby a poppy* produced at the control rate by the three normal talkers (N1, N2, N3) and the three apraxic talkers (A1, A2, A3). Because of disruptions in the syllabic pattern for some repetitions, the results for the apraxic speakers do not include all five repetitions. The tape-recorded model is represented by the filled bars.

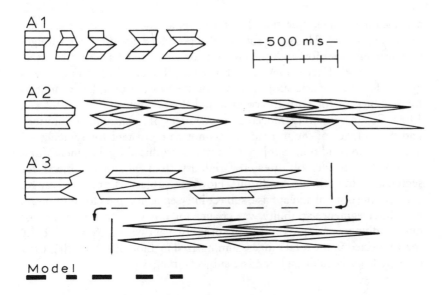

FIGURE 10-7. Temporal profiles for the pseudosyllables in *Build a big building* produced at the control rate by the apraxic subjects.

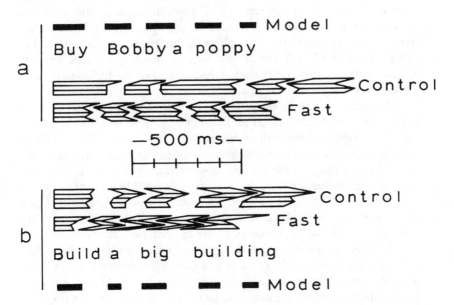

FIGURE 10-8. Temporal profiles for the pseudosyllables in *Buy Bobby a poppy* and *Build a big building*, produced by subject C2 at the two speaking rates.

average intersegment duration than the other apraxic subjects for sentence #1 at the fast rate. This same subject also produced a substantively longer intersegment duration with the fast rate for sentence #2 as did subject N1 for sentence #1. Intersegment variability for all data transformations was greater for the apraxic subjects than for the normal or aphasic subjects for sentence #1 for both the control and the fast rates (Tables 10-2 and 10-3). Group variability, reflected in the ranges of intersegment durations and percentages of the utterance, was not as consistent for sentence #2 at either rate condition. Subject A2 and A3 produced intersegment durations with considerably greater variability than all other subjects for sentence #2 in both rate conditions. However, subject A1 produced ranges closer to the normal and aphasic subject intersegment ranges for the control rate. Intersegment variability was greater for this subject during the fast rate condition and approximated the other two apraxic subjects' variability (best reflected in the total ranges, summarized in Table 10-5) which greatly exceeded the normal and aphasic subjects' ranges.

Intersegment-to-Segment Ratios

As a generality, the segment durations were longer than the intersegment durations for all subjects and all conditions. In several instances, however, the apraxic subjects produced average intersegment durations that were as long or longer than the segment durations (i.e., approached or exceeded a ratio of 1.0). The normal subjects never approached ratios of 1.0 and one aphasic subject approached a ratio of 1.0 for one utterance on sentence #2 for the fast rate.

The intersegment-to-segment ratios and trial-to-trial ranges for these ratios were considerably greater for the apraxic subjects than for the aphasic and normal subjects for both of the sentences in the control rate. Aphasic subject C1 produced an intersegment-to-segment ratio for sentence #1 that fell within the range of the apraxic subjects' ratios; however, it was based on only one production. The one average ratio for this particular conduction aphasic subject does, however, illustrate the general finding that their ratios were more variable from trial-to-trial than the normal subjects and overlapped with the large ranges of the apraxic subjects' ratios.

The fast rate produced a distribution of ratios similar to those of the control rate for each of the subjects and groups. Some of the apraxic subjects, on one of the sentences and one of the rate conditions, produced intersegment-to-segment ratios that were near or exceeded a ratio of 1.0 (i.e., 0.90–1.52). The normal subjects were less variable from trial to trial (total distribution of ratios ranged from 0.03 to 0.32 across sentences and rates) than the apraxic subjects (0.26–1.90) and the aphasic subjects (0.08–0.63).

Percentage of Segment and
Intersegment Change from Control to Fast Rate

Summarized in Tables 10-2 and 10-4 are the percentages of change that occurred with an increase of rate for each of the repeated sentences, for each subject, for the segment, and intersegment durations. Overall, the normal subjects reduced both their segment and intersegment durations to a greater degree than the apraxic or aphasic subjects. The apraxic subjects, in general, changed their segment and intersegment durations less than the normal subjects and less than the aphasic subjects. As with all other descriptive measures, however, there was considerable intrasubject variability between the two sentences. There was also great intersubject variability within groups. Apraxic subject #1 actually increased his segment durations by 3% in sentence #1 and his intersegment durations by 13% for sentence #2. Apraxic subject #2 increased his intersegment durations by 1% for sentence #1. All other changes were in the direction of reduced durations with increased rate. The conduction aphasic subjects' percentage of reduction generally approximated those of the normal subjects and were relatively equal between segment and intersegment reductions. No consistent patterns of change were identified for individuals or groups with respect to direction or amount of change from segment to intersegment durations other than the trend for the least change to occur for the apraxic subjects and the aphasic subjects' degree of change falling between the normal and apraxic subjects. As with all other measures, there was considerable intersubject overlap, both within and between groups. For example, subject A3 produced an intersegment duration reduction (Table 10-4) that approximated the greatest reduction of any of the normal subjects. Subject A2 produced the greatest reduction in segment durations for sentence #2 for the apraxic group, which approximated the greatest reduction in segment duration for the normal subjects. Again, the aphasic subjects tended to produce reduced durations that were between the values produced by the other two groups.

Voice Onset Time

A more detailed examination was made of the word *poppy* by determining durations for the acoustic–phonetic segments illustrated in Figure 10-3. The results are shown in Figure 10-9 for the three normal subjects, the three subjects with apraxia of speech, and the two subjects with conduction aphasia for whom measurements could be made. Generally, the temporal profiles for the five speakers with a neurologic disorder can be distinguished from those for the normal speakers in two primary ways: (1) lengthening of the total word duration and most of the component

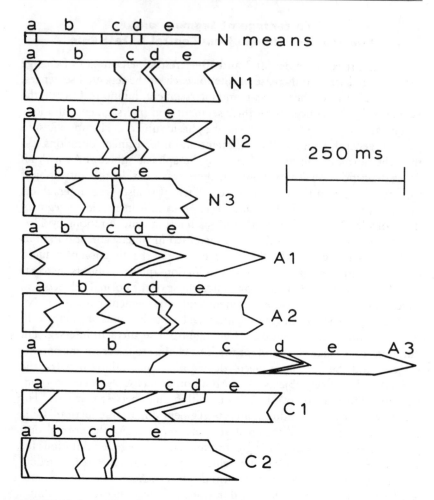

FIGURE 10-9. Temporal profiles for the acoustic-phonetic segments in the word *poppy* from *Buy Bobby a poppy* spoken at the control rate by all subjects. (a) voice onset time for the initial [p], (b) first syllable nucleus, (c) stop gap for [p], (d) voice onset time for second [p], and (e) second syllable nucleus.

segment durations; and (2) abnormalities of voice-onset time (VOT) for the word-initial [p]. Compared to the normal speakers, the subjects with apraxia of speech had longer and more variable VOTs for this sound. The two subjects with conduction aphasia showed divergent results for [p] VOT. Whereas C1 behaved like the apraxic subjects in having a longer VOT than the normal speakers, C2 had unusually short VOTs. These results indicate that abnormalities in the durations of acoustic–phonetic segments occur in the speech of both subjects with apraxia of speech and subjects with conduction aphasia.

Formant Trajectories

As a second closer look into the acoustic structure of the speech patterns of the normal and disordered speakers, we plotted the F2 (second formant) trajectories for the first syllable in the word *building*. Figure 10-10 shows the results for the three normal and the five disordered speakers. The five tracings of the trajectories for each normal speaker are quite similar, although the variability is not uniform among the three subjects. For N2, the tracings are nearly congruent, but a greater variability can be seen for N1 and N3. With the exception of A1, the F2 trajectories for the disordered speakers seem to be more variable than those for the normal speakers. Of particular importance is the fact that the trajectories for A2, A3, C1 and C2 differ not only in displacement along the frequency axis (as is the case for N3), but also in the temporal pattern of the trajectories. For example, particularly for A2 and C1, the patterns cannot be aligned simply by translation along the frequency or time axes.

DISCUSSION

The tentative conclusion we draw from our preliminary observations is that the nature of the disordered process in both apraxia of speech and conduction aphasia has phonetic and motoric components. We therefore use the term phonetic-motoric as a label for the impairment. However, this is not to say that apraxia of speech and conduction aphasia are one and the same impairment. They appear to strike at the phonetic-motoric realization of speech in different ways. With respect to the information-processing model in Figure 10-1, conduction aphasia appears to have its primary effect on phonetic coding and related or secondary effects on (1) working memory allocated to phonetic coding; and (2) motor control processes. Conduction aphasia may not seem to be a unitary disorder to the extent that the degree of impairment varies across phonetic coding, memory allocation, and motor control. Apraxia of speech seems to affect primarily motor control processes but has, perhaps consequentially, an effect on phonetic coding as well.

The model of Figure 10-1 is inadequate to represent speech production except in its most skeletal form. Eventually, the components labeled phonetic coding and motor control will have to be elaborated as, or replaced by, structures and processes such as those shown in Figure 10-2. For example, we think it is better to speak of prearticulatory representation

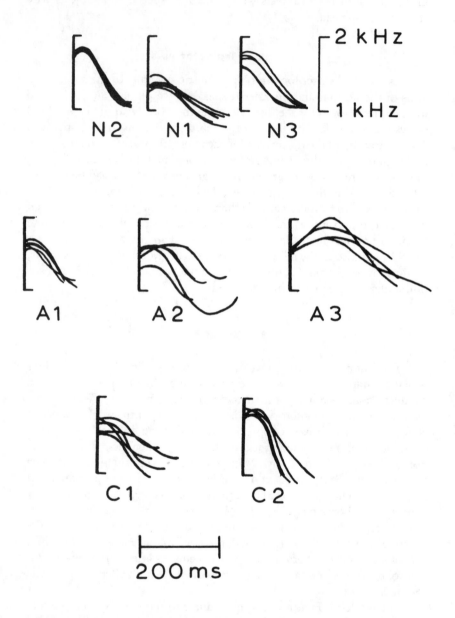

FIGURE 10-10. F2 (second formant) trajectories for pseudosyllable 4 in *Build a big building*. Data are shown for repetitions of this pseudosyllable by the three normal control subjects, the three apraxic subjects and two conduction aphasics.

than phonetic coding. The prearticulatory representation contains *slots and fillers* (Shattuck-Hufnagel, 1983) or *frames and contents* (MacNeilage, Studdert-Kennedy, & Lindblom, 1984). Slots-fillers and frames-contents are similar ideas about speech organization motivated largely by the conclusion that the explanation of normal speech sequencing errors, especially exchange errors, requires a separate specification of syllable structure and phonetic (or phonemic) segments. We believe that, at the least, the prearticulatory representation contains information on syllable structure and segment composition. Because these two bodies of information are held separately, they are susceptible to separate loss or error. Furthermore, the syllabic and segmental specifications only gradually lose their separateness in motor control. Syllabic organization is a primary level of cohesion in which, (1) suprasegmental information is given form in the prosodic envelope of a syllabic sequence; and (2) segmental information is converted to movements (preferably compound trajectories defined by compatible sequential goals [Shaffer, 1982]). Finally, the prosodic envelope based on syllabic sequences guides output monitoring and is a first line of linkage between the monitored acoustic output and the slot-filler specifications in the prearticulatory representation. When phonetic-motoric coding is vulnerable to error, as in the neurologic disorders studied here, speakers may allocate more resources to the slot-filler specifications of individual syllables and their motoric realization. Syllable lengthening and long intersyllabic pauses may result.

Our observations of speech production in conduction aphasia do not accord fully with descriptions in the literature. In particular, we present preliminary evidence that this disorder is not a monolithic phonologic-level disturbance. The abnormalities in segment and intersegment durations, voice onset time, and formant trajectories are best interpreted as meaning that motoric planning, or execution, or both, are disrupted. To be sure, a larger set of acoustic or physiological data are needed to substantiate this interpretation. But our observations at least open the door to the working hypothesis that conduction aphasia is characterized by frequent phonemic paraphasias *and* speech abnormalities at the phonetic-motoric level. In this respect, conduction aphasia is similar to apraxia of speech, which originally was considered as having predominantly substitutions and other phonemic-level errors, but more recently is viewed by several investigators as affecting motor timing and coordination (see review in Rosenbek et al., 1984).

Conduction aphasia rarely has come under a close acoustic or physiologic analysis. Most reports are based on auditory phonetic descriptions. Given the perceptual salience of phonemic paraphasias, it is not surprising that these highly conspicuous errors dominated the clinical descriptions of this disorder. But the question we pose is whether it is sufficient to consider only phonemic-level errors in the understanding of conduction aphasia.

The co-occurrence of phonemic paraphasias with phonetic or motoric abnormalities raises some interesting theoretical questions. For example, are there really two kinds of disruption—one phonemic and the other phonetic-motoric—or are both of these manifestations of a common underlying disorder? One interpretation is that disruptions in phonological processing or phonetic realization have motoric consequences in the form of abnormal temporal patterns. That is, uncertainties or inefficiencies at a relatively abstract level of speech are reflected in the motor processes that they drive. Another interpretation is that the theoretical division between phonetic representation and motor realization is invalid. Instead of supposing that these are two different levels related by an intervening process, they might be viewed as being fundamentally inseparable. Phonetic representation is accomplished in terms of motoric prescriptions. This idea is similar to that expressed by proponents of action theory.

It was characteristic of the apraxic subjects we studied to have a slow speaking rate manifested as increased durations of pseudosyllable segments and the intervals between them. Slow speaking rate can result from several factors, including motoric limitations, compensation for motoric difficulties, or an attempt to reinstall effective self-monitoring. Each or all of these factors could be involved in apraxia of speech. Further insight into the disorder can be achieved by a more detailed consideration of the data. First, the apraxic speakers appear to differ from the other speakers, both normal subjects and conduction aphasics, in having large intersegment intervals. These long intervals between pseudosyllables were essentially uniformly distributed in the sentence repetitions, as can be seen in Figures 10-6 and 10-7. Although the conduction aphasics also had frequent interruptions within a sentence repetition, the interruptions were not so regularly distributed as they were for the apraxic subjects. The conduction aphasic was more likely to produce a few syllables with an essentially normal tempo but then interrupt the syllable sequence with a long pause. The occurrence of such occasional interruptions in conduction aphasia thus appears different from the disturbance of speech flow typical of the apraxic subjects.

Apraxic speakers and conduction aphasics were similar in some respects and different in others. Both groups produced a number of speech errors that would be described clinically as substitutions. The frequent appearance of this kind of error in both disorders has been a primary reason for their classification by some writers as phonologic disorders. Substitutions, intrusions, and omissions are ostensibly the results of operations on phoneme-sized units and it is tempting therefore to regard these errors as evidence for phonological impairment.

But apraxia of speech is characterized by more than phonemic errors, no matter how much the phonemic level may have dominated early descriptions of the disorder. The overall speech pattern is typically slow and, as already noted, rather regularly interrupted by intersyllabic pauses. Apraxia of speech has a conspicuous dysprosody, although it is not clear if the dysprosody is an independent feature of the disorder or simply a consequence of a primary articulatory impairment. Our results indicate that apraxic speakers are not particularly successful at managing changes in speaking rate. Sometimes, an attempted production at a fast rate actually yielded an overall utterance duration longer than that observed for control rate productions. Difficulty in rate management seems to point to a motoric inflexibility in the apraxic speaker.

Conduction aphasia does not share with apraxia of speech a pervasive dysprosody. Over short intervals, the conduction aphasics had an essentially normal prosodic pattern. Furthermore, the conduction aphasics were much more successful than the apraxic speakers in managing changes in speaking rate. This is not to say that conduction aphasics are not challenged by increased rate of speech. It was our impression that their phonemic or phonetic errors increased in number as rate of speaking increased. However, unlike the apraxic speakers, the subjects with conduction aphasia could increase syllabic rate and in this respect the conduction aphasics seem to retain a motoric flexibility that is lost in apraxia of speech.

Our data are preliminary and cannot be the basis for sweeping conclusions about these complex and perplexing disorders. We hope that we have pointed the way to analyses that hold the potential for increased understanding. In particular, we suggest that the methods of acoustic analysis can lead to refined descriptions of the speech abnormalities in these disorders that seem to affect both phonologic and motoric processing. It may be that a sharp distinction between these two levels of processing is not justified. Most writers who have favored one level over the other as the primary aspect of disruption have based their conclusions on data obtained at one level only, thus confusing conclusion with analysis method.

Variability

The paradigm governing research in aphasia since the early 1860's has been, and continues to be the centers and pathways models of brain function. In short, the centers and pathways models of aphasia state that there are specific centers in the brain (primarily the left-hemisphere cortex and possibly subcortex) that house specific linguistic functions and are connected to one another via pathways that transmit information from center-to-center for formulation, concatenation, elaboration, or execution. The centers and pathways models are most often attributed in origin to Wernicke and Lictheim but they have been modernized and popularized by such contemporary American aphasiologists as Geschwind, Benson, and Goodglass. According to these models, a lesion in either a "language" center or a pathway connecting two critical centers will cause a specific and predictable aphasic syndrome. These models and the classification systems that they have spawned have come under considerable criticism of late. The criticisms have ranged from the probability of misapplying therapeutic principles because of the heterogeneity of subjects within any type of aphasia (Darley, 1982), to the failure of such classifications to inform neuropsychological–cognitive theories of aphasia (Caramazza, 1984), to the classifications systems' invalidity on a construct level (McNeil, 1984), to the inability of the centers and pathways models to account for the variable performance that is a hallmark of aphasic behavior (McNeil, 1982). With few exceptions, the explanations offered for the item to item or moment to moment speech and language variability in aphasic performance have been attributed to changes among the stimuli used to evoke the response. In many cases, these linguistic, motoric or communicative variables do in fact predict, with a high degree of accuracy, the performance of the aphasic or apraxic subject. In these instances, the pathologic behavior is attributed to a focal lesion within a language center or in a pathway connecting two or more centers, as depicted in Figure 10-3. However, a simple center lesion or a disconnection explanation does not appear to offer a satisfactory account of the trial-to-trial variability on the exact same utterance produced under identical motoric and communicative conditions. This variability best typifies the pathological subjects' performance across all of the acoustic analyses in this investigation. The apraxic and aphasic subjects, on occasion, produced a particular segment, intersegment, VOT or second formant of an utterance, even if on only 1 in 5 trials, within the limits of the normal subjects. The neuroanatomic and linguistic models proposed thus far, including the centers and pathways models do not satisfactorily address this component of the pathological mechanism. The model offered in Figure 10-1, likewise, does not address this moment-to-moment variability. Perhaps something akin to the attention, resource allocation and fluctuating biological rhythms mechanisms proposed by McNeil (1982, 1983) and McNeil and Kimelman (1986) to account for the variability of the auditory processing and comprehension system, will eventually explain this source of variability in the speech and language of the aphasic and the apraxic person. Perhaps the model proposed in Figure 10-1 and those developed to account for various aspects of the phonetic and linguistic systems of the neurologically impaired will require the incorporation of a resource allocation component, or other, as yet undiscovered construct that will address the moment-to-moment variability that characterizes apraxic and aphasic behavior at all linguistic and motoric levels.

ACKNOWLEDGMENT

This work was supported by Public Health Service research grants NS18797 and NS22458.

REFERENCES

Blumstein, S.E., Cooper, W.E., Goodglass, H., Statlender, S., & Gottlieb, J. (1980). Production deficits in aphasia: A voice-onset-time analysis. *Brain and Language*, 9, 153–170.

Bock, J.K. (1982). Toward a cognitive psychology of syntax: Information processing contribution to sentence formulation. *Psychological Review*, 89, 1–47.

Boomer, D.S., & Laver, J.D. (1968). Slips of the tongue. *British Journal of Disorders of Communication*, 3, 2–12.

Borkowski, J.G., Benton, A.L., & Spreen, O. (1967). Word fluency and brain damage. *Neuropsychologia*, 5, 135–140.

Brown, J.W. (1975). The problem of repetition: a study of "conduction" aphasia and the "isolation" syndrome. *Cortex*, 11, 37–52.

Brown, R., & McNeill, D. (1966). The "tip of the tongue" phenomenon. *Journal of Verbal Learning and Verbal Behavior*, 5, 325–327.

Butterworth, B. (1979). Hesitation and the production of verbal paraphasias and neologisms in jargon aphasia. *Brain and Language*, 8, 133–161.

Caramazza, A. (1984). The logic of neuropsychological research and the problem of patient classification in aphasia. *Brain and Language*, 21, 9–20.

Carlson, R., & Granstrom, B. (1986). A search for durational rates in a real-speech data base. *Phonetica*, 43, 140–154.

Chafe, W.L. (1977). Creativity in verbalization and its implication for the nature of stored knowledge. In R.O. Freedle (Ed.), *Discourse production and comprehension* (Vol. 1). Norwood, NJ: Ablex.

Chomsky, N. (1965). *Aspects of the theory of syntax*. Cambridge, MA: MIT Press.

Chomsky, N., & Halle, M. (1968). *The sound pattern of english*. New York: Harper and Row.

Crystal, T.H., & House, A.S. (1982). Segmented durations in connected speech signals: Preliminary results. *Journal of the Acoustical Society of America*, 72, 705–716.

Dabul, B. (1979). *Apraxia battery for adults*. Tigard, OR: C.C. Publications.

Damasio, H., & Damasio, A. (1980). The anatomical basis of conduction aphasia, *Brain*, 103, 337–350.

Darley, F.L. (1982). *Aphasia*. New York: Saunders.

Darley, F., Aronson, A., & Brown, J. (1975). *Motor speech disorders*. Philadelphia: Saunders.

Dubois, J., Hecaen, H., Angelengues, R., de Chatelier, A., & Marcie, P. (1964). Etude neurolinguistique de l'aphasie de conduction. *Neuropsychologia*, 2, 9–44. Translated in H. Goodglass & S.E. Blumstein (Eds.), *Psycholinguistics and aphasia*, Baltimore: Johns Hopkins Press, 1973.

Ford, M., & Holmes, V.M. (1978). Planning units and syntax in sentence production. *Cognition*, 6, 35–53.

Fowler, C., Rubin, P., Remez, R.E., & Turvey, M.T. (1980). Implications for speech production of a general theory of action. In B. Butterworth (Ed.), *Speech production* (Vol. 1). New York: Academic Press.

Friedrich, F.J., Glenn, C.G., & Marin, O.S.M. (1984). Interruption of phonological coding in conduction aphasia. *Brain and Language*, 22, 266–291.

Fromkin, V.A. (1966). Neuromuscular specification of linguistic units. *Language and Speech, 9,* 170–199.

Fromkin, V.A. (1973). Slips of the tongue. *Scientific American, 229,* 110–117.

Garney, S.M., & Dell, G.S. (1984). Some neurolinguistic implications of prearticulatory editing in speech production. *Brain and Language, 23,* 64–73.

Garrett, M.R. (1980). Levels of processing in sentence production. In B. Butterworth (Ed.), *Language production* (Vol. 1). London: Academic Press.

Gee, J.P., & Grosjean, F. (1983). Performance structure: A psycho-linguistic and linguistic appraisal. *Cognitive Psychology, 15,* 411–458.

Geschwind, N. (1965). Disconnection syndromes in animals and man. *Brain, 88,* 237–274, 585–644.

Goodglass, H. (1983). Word retrieval for production. In M. Studdert-Kennedy (Ed.), *Psychobiology of language.* Cambridge, Mass: MIT Press.

Goodglass, H., & Kaplan, E. (1983). *Boston diagnostic aphasia examination* (2nd Ed.). Philadelphia: Lea Febiger.

Henke, W.L. (1966). Dynamic articulatory model of speech production using computer simulation (Unpublished doctoral dissertation, Massaschusetts Institute of Technology, Cambridge, Massachusetts).

Jakobson, R., Fant, C.G.M., & Halle, M. (1951). *Preliminaries to speech analysis: The distinctive features and their correlates.* Cambridge, MA: MIT Press.

Kelso, J.A.S., Tuller, B., & Harris, K.S. (1983). A "dynamic pattern" perspective on the control and coordination of movement. In P.F. MacNeilage (Ed.), *The production of speech.* New York: Springer-Verlag.

✓ Kempen, G., & Huijbers, P. (1983). The lexicalization process in sentence production and naming: Indirect election of words. *Cognition, 14,* 185–209.

Kent, R.D. (1984). Brain mechanisms of speech and language with special reference to emotional interactions. In R. Naremose (Ed.), *Language science: Recent advances.* San Diego: College-Hill Press.

Kent, R.D., Carney, P.J., & Severeid, L.R. (1974). Velar movement and timing: Evaluation of a model for binary control. *Journal of Speech and Hearing Research, 17,* 470–488.

Kent, R.D., & Rosenbek, J.C. (1983). Acoustic patterns of apraxia of speech. *Journal of Speech and Hearing Research, 26,* 231–248.

Kohn, S.E. (1984). The nature of the phonological disorder in conduction aphasia. *Brain and Language, 23,* 97–115.

Kozhevnikov, V.A., & Chistovich, L.A. (1965). *Speech: Articulation and perception.* Washington, DC: U.S. Government Printing Office.

Ladefoged, P., Declerk, J., Lindau, M., & Papcun, G. (1972). An auditory-motor theory of speech production. *UCLA Working Papers in Linguistics, 22,* 48–75.

Lesser, R. (1978). *Linguistic investigations of aphasia.* London: Arnold.

Levelt, W.J.M. (1983). Monitoring and self-repair in speech. *Cognition, 14,* 41–104.

Liberman, A.M. (1970). The grammars of language and speech. *Cognitive Psychology, 1,* 301–323.

Liberman, A.M., Cooper, F.J., Shankweiler, D.P., & Studdert-Kennedy, M. (1967). Perception of the speech code. *Psychological Review, 74,* 431–461.

Lichtenstein, E.H., & Brewer, W.F. (1980). Memory for goal-directed events. *Cognitive Psychology, 12,* 412–445.

Lindblom, B., Lubker, J., & Gay, T. (1979). Formant frequencies of some fixed-mandible vowels and a model of speech motor programming by predictive simulation. *Journal of Phonetics, 7*, 147–161.

Lindsley, J.R. (1975). Producing simple utterances: How far ahead do we plan? *Cognitive Psychology, 7*, 1–19.

Lindsley, J.R. (1976). Producing simple utterances: Details of the planning process. *Journal of Psycholinguistics, 5*, 331–354.

Lynch, J.J. (1985). *The Language of the heart.* New York: Basic Books.

MacKay, D.G. (1974). Aspects of the symbol of behavior: Syllable structure and speech rate. *Quarterly Journal of Experimental Psychology, 26*, 642–657.

MacNeilage, P.F. (1970). Motor control of serial ordering of speech. *Psychological Review, 77*, 182–196.

MacNeilage, P.F., Studdert-Kennedy, M., & Lindblom, B. (1984). Functional precursors to language and its lateralization. *American Journal of Physiology, 246 (Regulatory Integrative and Comparative Physiology, 15)*, R912–R914.

McCarthy, R., & Warrington, E.K. (1984). A two-route model of speech production: Evidence from aphasia. *Brain, 107*, 463–485.

McNeil, M.R. (1982). The nature of aphasia in adults. In: N J. Lass, L.V. McReynolds, J.L. Northern, & D.E. Yoder, (Eds.), *Speech, language and hearing: Vol II. Speech and language pathology.* Philadelphia: W.B. Saunders.

McNeil, M.R. (1983). Aphasia: Neurological considerations. *Topics in Language Disorders, 3*(4), 1–19.

McNeil, M.R. (1984). Current concepts in adult aphasia. *International Rehabilitative Medicine, 6*, 128–134.

McNeil, M.R., & Kimelman, D.D.Z. (1986). Toward an integrative information-processing structure of auditory comprehension and processing in adult aphasia. *Seminars in Speech and Language, 7*(2), 123–146.

McNeil, M.R., & Prescott, T.E. (1978). *Revised token test.* Baltimore: University Park Press.

Mermelstein, P. (1973). Articulatory model for the study of speech production. *Journal of the Acoustical Society of America, 53*, 1070–1082.

Meyer, D.E., & Gordon, P.C. (1985). Speech production: Motor programming of phonetic features. *Journal of Memory and Language, 24*, 3–26.

Miller, J.L., Grosjean, F., & Lomanto, C. (1984). Articulation rate and its variability in spontaneous speech: A reanalysis and some implications. *Phonetica, 41*, 215–225.

Mlcoch, A.G., & Noll, J.D. (1980). Speech production models as related to the concept of apraxia of speech. In N.J. Lass (Ed.), *Speech and language: Advances in basic research and practice.* New York: Academic Press.

Nolan, F.J. (1982). The role of action theory in the description of speech production. *Linguistics, 20*, 287–308.

O'Connell, P.F. (1981). Neologistic jargon aphasia: A case report. *Brain and Language, 12*, 292–302.

Porch, B.E. (1967). *Porch index of communicative ability.* Palo Alto, CA: Consulting Psychologists Press.

Raven, J.C. (1962). *Coloured progressive materials.* London: H.K. Lewis.

Reed, E.S. (1982). An outline of a theory of action systems. *Journal of Motor Behavior*, 14, 98–134.

Rosenbaum, D.A., Weber, R.J., Hazellett, W.M., & Hindorff, V. (1986). The parameter remapping effect in human performance: Evidence from tongue twisters and finger fumbles. *Journal of Memory and Language*, 25, 710–725.

Rosenbek, J.C., Kent, R.D., & LaPointe, L.L. (1984). Apraxia of speech: An overview and some perspectives. In J.C. Rosenbek, M.R. McNeil, & A. Aronson (Eds.), *Apraxia of speech: Physiology, acoustics, linguistics and management*. San Diego: College-Hill Press.

Schank, R. (1972). Conceptual dependency: A theory of natural language understanding. *Cognitive Psychology*, 3, 552–631.

Seinsch, W. (1981). Artikulatorische dyspraxie. *Folia Phoniatrica*, 33, 125–130.

Shaffer, L.H. (1982). Rhythm and timing in skill. *Psychological Review*, 89, 109–122.

Shallice, T., & Warrington, E.K. (1977). Auditory-verbal short-term memory impairment and conduction aphasia. *Brain and Language*, 4, 479–491.

Shattuck-Hufnagel, S. (1983). Sublexical units and suprasegmental structure in speech production planning. In P.F. MacNeilage (Ed.), *The Production of speech*. New York: Springer-Verlag.

Shattuck-Hufnagel, S., & Klatt, D.H. (1979). The limited use of distinctive features and markedness in speech production: Evidence from speech error data. *Journal of Verbal Learning and Verbal Behavior*, 18, 41–55.

Sternberg, S., Monsell, S., Knoll, R.L., & Wright, C.E. (1978). The latency and duration of rapid movement sequences: Comparison of speech and typewriting. In G.E. Stelmach (Ed.), *Information processing in motor control and learning*. New York: Academic Press.

Tatham, M.A.A. (1970). A speech production model for synthesis-by-rule. *Working papers in linguistics*, (Vol. 6). Ohio State University: Computer and Information Sciences Research Center.

Warrington, E.K., Logue, V., & Pratt, R.T.C. (1971). The anatomical localization of selective impairment of auditory verbal short term memory. *Neuropsychologia*, 9, 377–387.

Warrington, E.K., & Shallice, T. (1972). Neuropsychological evidence of visual storage in short-term memory tasks. *Quarterly Journal of Experimental Psychology*, 24, 30–40.

Weismer, G., & Fennel, A.M. (1985). Constancy of (acoustic) relative timing measures in phrase-level utterances. *Journal of the Acoustical Society of America*, 78, 49–57.

Wickelgren, W.A. (1969). Content-sensitive coding, associative memory, and serial order in (speech) behavior. *Psychological Review*, 76, 1–15.

Yamadori, A., & Ikumura, G. (1975). Central (or conduction) aphasia in a Japanese patient. *Cortex*, 11, 73–82.

C H A P T E R   11

Anticipatory Labial and Lingual Coarticulation in Aphasia

William F. Katz

The study of anticipatory (or *right-to-left*) coarticulation is of special interest to speech researchers because it is considered to be a measure of the *preplanning* of upcoming speech segments. By examining speakers' ability to anticipate articulatory configurations it is possible to gain insight into the size and nature of motor sequencing units, as well as their control.

Two of the most widely studied forms of anticipatory coarticulation are anticipatory *labial* and *lingual* coarticulation. Anticipatory labial coarticulation involves the initiation of a rounding gesture during consonant production preceding a rounded vowel. For example, a speaker producing the English syllable [tu] will round his lips at the start of the [t] in anticipation of the rounded vowel [u]. In contrast, no rounding occurs when he is producing the syllable [ti]. Anticipatory coarticulation has been studied by a variety of articulatory, acoustic and perceptual methods. Articulatory studies have indicated that anticipatory labialization reliably occurs in a number of languages, and that the timing and extent of these gestures are language-particular (see Ohde & Sharf, 1981; Lubker & Gay, 1982, for reviews). Acoustic investigations using spectrographic and Linear Predictive Coding (LPC) analyses have shown that there are systematic acoustic correlates for anticipatory labialization in both stop-vowel (Ohman, 1966; Fant, 1973; Sereno et al., 1987) and fricative-vowel (Soli, 1981; Sereno et al., 1987) syllables. In addition, it has been established that labial coarticulatory information may be reliably detected by listeners. For example, studies have shown that subjects, given only a short duration aperiodic section of the preceding consonantal segment, are able to correctly identify the missing vowel of stop-vowel (Winitz, Scheib, & Reeds, 1972; LaRiviere, Winitz, & Herriman, 1975a; Ohde & Sharf, 1977; Sereno et al., 1987) and fricative-vowel (LaRiviere, Winitz & Herriman, 1975b; Yeni-Komshian & Soli, 1981; Sereno et al., 1987) CV stimuli.

Anticipatory lingual coarticulation involves the front and back positioning of the tongue in velar stop closure as a function of the feature specification of the following vowel. For example, in English, the phoneme /k/ has a front allophone with a relatively anterior vocal tract constriction, and a back allophone with a relatively posterior constriction. This difference in the point of oral cavity constriction corresponds with robust spectral differences between front and back allophones of /k/ (Potter, Kopp, & Green, 1947; Halle, Hughes, & Radley, 1957; Zue, 1976). Perceptual experiments in which listeners are given excised prevocalic velar stop stimuli have demonstrated that context-dependent information is clearly present in brief portions of these stimuli (Schatz, 1954; Winitz et al., 1972; Lieberman & Sereno, 1986).

COARTICULATION AND APHASIA

Traditional clinical descriptions of aphasia consider the errors in speech produced by posterior (Wernicke's) aphasics to originate at the phoneme planning level whereas phonetic or articulatory errors are thought to be more typical of anterior, nonfluent aphasia (Alajouanine, Ombredane, & Durand, 1939; Luria, 1966). In recent years, fine-grained acoustic analyses have uncovered additional data that generally support this dichotomy, although a number of studies suggest that the Wernicke's aphasics may exhibit subtle phonetic deficits that are not clinically evident (Blumstein, et al., 1977; Tuller, 1984; Ryalls, 1986). Studies supporting this phonetic–phonemic deficit dichotomy have examined various aspects of segmental units in aphasic speech production, including voice onset time (VOT) of consonants (Blumstein et al., 1977; Blumstein, et al., 1980; Shewan, Leeper & Booth, 1984; Gandour & Dardarananda, 1984) and the duration (Peterson & Lehiste, 1960; Tikofsky, 1965; Ryalls, 1982, 1986), formant frequencies, and fundamental frequency of vowels (Ryalls, 1984; 1986). The general picture that has emerged with respect to anterior aphasics is that these subjects have impairments in the timing or integration of movements of the articulatory system. This has been referred to as "the reduction of the capacity for independent movement of the articulators" (Shankweiler & Harris, 1966), "deficits in temporal control" (Freeman, Sands, & Harris, 1978), "poor temporal control" (Sands, Freeman, & Harris, 1978), "disturbance of time programming for articulation" (Itoh, Sasanuma, & Ushijima, 1979) and "aberrant phase relationships in hetero-organic speech gestures" (Ziegler & von Cramon, 1985).

It has been further hypothesized that anterior aphasics demonstrate impairments in laryngeal control and in the timing of two independent articulators (Blumstein et al., 1977; 1980; Freeman et al., 1978; Itoh et al., 1979; Shewan et al., 1984; Gandour & Dardarananda, 1984), rather than global impairments in the coordination of articulatory movements, e.g., getting the vocal tract into the appropriate configuration for place of articulation in stop consonants (Shinn & Blumstein, 1983).

The majority of studies exploring these hypotheses have focussed upon speech production at the level of individual sounds and have not addressed *sound transitional* or coarticulatory phenomena. However, recent investigations have pointed out the importance of examining coarticulatory phenomena in aphasia as a possible key to understanding the speech motor deficits of these subjects. Ziegler and von Cramon (1985) measured the degree of labial anticipatory coarticulation in read CVCVC utterances produced by a German-speaking apraxia of speech subject. Based upon listeners' identification scores for postconsonantal vowels when given gated portions of the preceding consonant, the authors concluded that this subject showed a "delayed onset of anticipatory vowel gestures relative to the labial occlusion." In a subsequent acoustic experiment, Ziegler and von Cramon (1986a) measured vowel-to-vowel and vowel-to-consonant anticipatory coarticulation in the speech of this same patient by means of formant frequency and LP reflection coefficient analyses. The results, which largely hinged on the formant frequency data and much less on the LP reflection coefficient data, were also considered to reveal "a consistent delay in the initiation of vowel gestures" in the speech of this subject. Ziegler and von Cramon (1986b) extended this type of acoustic analysis to include data from 5 additional apraxia of speech subjects. LP reflection coefficients for burst spectra of prevocalic [t] produced by normal and verbal apraxic subjects were entered into a discriminant analysis. For productions by normal speakers, 98% of the rounded and unrounded tokens were correctly classified, whereas there was 72% correct classification for the verbal apraxic subjects' productions. These data were considered to support the notion of a deficiency in anticipatory coarticulation in the speech of verbal apraxic subjects.

Tuller and Story (1986) analyzed coarticulatory information in LPC-derived spectra of the fricative portion of FVC stimuli produced by 5 fluent and 5 non-fluent aphasics. The authors found that normal control subjects' spectral peaks varied with the postconsonantal vowel, as did the spectral peaks of the productions by the fluent aphasics. In contrast, only one nonfluent speaker showed evidence of anticipatory or carryover coarticulation. These results suggested a possible deficit in anticipatory coarticulation in the speech of nonfluent aphasics.

The present investigation was designed to explore in detail whether anterior aphasic subjects, in addition to evidencing timing problems at the *segmental* level, show sound-transitional (*phasing* or coarticulatory) deficits. Two experiments are described that assessed anticipatory coarticulation in CV and CCV stimuli produced by anterior and posterior aphasics. In the first experiment, acoustic correlates of anticipatory labial and lingual coarticulation are analyzed by means of LPC analysis. In the second experiment, a subset of the consonantal stimuli produced by the normal and aphasic subjects were given to a group of naive listeners for a vowel identification task. Based on the data of Ziegler and von Cramon (1985, 1986a, 1986b) and Tuller and Story (1986), it might be expected that anterior aphasics would show coarticulatory deficits in CV and CCV productions. If anterior aphasics show coarticulatory deficits this would have important consequences for neurolinguistic theories which hold, for example, that Broca's area is specialized for "speech motor programming" (e.g., Luria, 1966; Darley, Aronson, & Brown, 1975; Mlcoch & Noll, 1980). Conversely, if anterior aphasics do not show coarticulatory impairments, this would suggest that patients with cortical damage to pre-Rolandic tissue retain a greater degree of intact timing capacities than previously expected.

A second and related question is whether Wernicke's aphasics show anticipatory coarticulation deficits. Since labial anticipatory coarticulatory effects do not reflect phonological contrasts in English, on the model that Wernicke's aphasics exhibit a primarily phonological planning problem, one would expect their coarticulatory patterns to be unimpaired. However, given that Wernicke's aphasics also appear to have a subtle phonetic deficit, it might also be the case that this deficit involves coarticulatory preplanning. If this is the case, then Wernicke's aphasics might also show anticipatory coarticulation impairments.

ACOUSTIC EXPERIMENT

Subjects

The aphasic subject population consisted of 5 anterior and 5 posterior aphasics. The subjects were right-handed males who had acquired aphasia as the result of stroke. All subjects were naive speakers of English, with no known history of hearing loss. The average of the aphasic patients was 60.1 years (SD = 10.3), 61.8 for anteriors, and 58.4 for posteriors. Patients' clinical classification, lesion site, and time between onset of aphasia and testing are described in detail in Katz (1987). Four of the subjects were outpatients of the Speech Therapy Ward of Long Beach VA Hospital, and the remaining 6 subjects were out-patients of the Aphasia Ward of the Boston VA Medical Center.

The language and speech characteristics of the aphasic patients were assessed using the Boston Diagnostic Aphasia Examination (Goodglass & Kaplan, 1972), and by clinical examination. Patients were assigned to aphasic groups on the basis of both clinical exam and lesion localization, as well as the consensus of the neurologists, psychologists, and speech pathologists at the aphasia rounds of both the Boston VA Aphasia Center and Long Beach VA Speech Therapy Center. All of the anterior aphasia subjects fit the description of Broca's aphasia, as defined by the BDAE classification system. In addition to their aphasic impairments, two of the anterior subjects, A4 and A5, were also described as having speech distortions characteristic of dysarthria (cf. Katz, 1987). All of the posterior aphasic subjects could be classified as Wernicke's aphasics, with the exception of P3. This patient, who had a large parietal lesion, presented with grammatically fluent speech, yet was described as showing "moderate apraxia of speech" characterized by delayed initiation, groping, and searching for correct articulatory positions. Subject P4 may be termed a *recovered Wernicke's aphasic*, in that this subject presented with expressive characteristics typical of Wernicke's aphasia, yet had recovered a good degree of auditory comprehension skills. The initial BDAE auditory comprehension scores for this subject were − 0.5.

Six adult males from the Boston University community volunteered as control subjects. The average age of this (nonage-matched) control group was 27.8 years old (SD = 7.3 years).

Stimuli

Subjects were asked to read the following words and nonsense-syllables:

see [si]	sue [su]
tea [ti]	two [tu]
key [ki]	coo [ku]
"stee" [sti]	stew]stu]
ski [ski]	"skoo" [sku]

These words were printed individually on 3 × 5 index cards in large type. The two nonsense syllables were indicated with quotation marks. Stimuli were presented to subjects 10 times, in a single randomized order. If an aphasic patient could not read a word, he was asked to repeat it after the investigator. In this event, care was taken by the investigator to conceal his lips in order to prevent imitation of labial gestures.

Acoustic Analysis

Analysis focussed on the initial fricative and stop in CV stimuli, and on the initial fricative in CCV stimuli. The voiceless consonants [s], [t], and [k] were selected for analysis because there are previous data for these items with respect to labial and lingual anticipatory coarticulation effects (Soli, 1981; Lieberman & Sereno, 1986; Sereno et al., 1987). Consonant cluster-vowel syllables ([stV] and [skV]) were included as stimuli in order to explore whether acoustic correlates of anticipatory coarticulation of the vowel would emerge in the production of [s] across an intervening stop consonant. In addition, it is known that consonant cluster stimuli are some of the most difficult items for aphasic subjects to produce (Blumstein, 1973). Hence, the inclusion of consonant cluster stimuli also allows an investigation of whether anticipatory coarticulation in aphasia varies as a function of the "difficulty" of the consonantal sequence.

Subjects' speech was transcribed phonetically from audio tapes by the investigator. Instances of aphasic subjects' phonemic substitution and articulatory errors (e.g., prolonged [s], heavy aspiration of consonant) were noted and discarded (cf. Katz, 1987). The resulting stimuli were analyzed on a PDP 11/34 computer at the Brown University Phonetics Laboratory, using the WAVED speech-analysis program (Mertus, 1980). Tokens were digitized and the waveform of each stimulus was visually displayed for editing on a monitor.

Consonantal segments were identified using the following criteria: for the [s] of the [sV] utterances, cursors were placed at the start and end of the frication noise to isolate that portion of the speech signal independent of vocalic transition and vowel. The start of the frication noise was identified as the first visibly noticeable turbulence in the waveform. The end of frication was defined as the portion of the noise immediately preceding the start of vocalic transition. For the [s] portion of the [stV] and [skV] utterances, the same criteria were used to define the start of frication noise. The end of frication was defined as the portion of noise preceding the silence corresponding to the closure for the subsequent [t] or [k] stop. For the stop consonant stimuli, the aperiodic portion of the signal was defined as that portion including the release and aspiration noise.

Spectra of the aperiodic segments corresponding to the intitial consonant of each stimulus were obtained using computer-implemented fourier analysis and 24-term LPC (Rabiner & Schafter, 1979). For each stimulus, a 20 ms window was placed over *early* and *late* regions of the initial consonantal waveform. In each case, the *late* region was defined as the final 20 ms of the initial consonantal segment. The exact location of the *early* region differed with consonant type. For [s], the *early* region was defined as being 70 ms prior to the onset of the vowel transition. For the initial stop consonants [t] and [k], the *early* region was defined as the initial 20 ms of the waveform, i.e., the release. An example of a waveform for [si] produced by one of the normal subjects is given in Figure 11-1. Cursors (labeled L1, R1) mark the beginning and end of the fricative [s]. A 20 ms full Hamming LPC window is placed over the *early* and *late* regions of the waveform.

Two spectral prominence regions (*low* and *high*) were measured in order to assess the presence of coarticulation. The *low* frequency region corresponds to the starting frequency of the second formant of the vowel. Consistent coarticulatory shift in this frequency region has been observed by a number of researchers (Soli, 1981; Turnbaugh, Hoffman, & Daniloff,

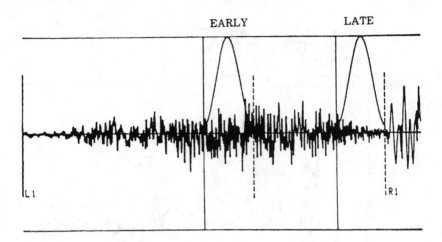

EARLY   LATE

L 1   R 1

FIGURE 11-1. Waveform display of [si].

1985; Sereno et al., 1987). The *high* frequency region corresponds to peaks which have been observed in [s] and [t] spectra (cf. Katz, 1987, for details). these *high* frequency peaks will henceforth also be referred to as the "characteristic spectral prominence" (CSP) for the consonant.

Spectral peaks were determined by a two-stage procedure. First, *low* and *high* frequency regions were visually determined from superimposed LPC plots of each subject's repeated productions. The next step involved selecting, for each token, the peak frequency values located within these prespecified frequency regions. These values were taken directly from the (numeric) output of the LPC program. If multiple peaks occurred within a frequency region, the highest amplitude peak was chosen.

Figure 11-2 shows the spectrum for the *late* window of [si] (solid line) and [su] (dotted line) produced by speaker N1. The peaks located within *low* and *high* frequency regions are indicated with arrows. It will be observed that the [su] spectrum is "shifted" down in frequency by approximately 300 Hz. This shift and, in particular, the shift in the second formant and CSP frequency regions, constitutes the dependent variables for the labial anticipatory coarticulation stimuli, i.e., formant lowering associated with lengthening of the vocal tract by labial rounding.

In the case of the velar stimuli, [kV], context-dependent spectral differences are even greater than for the other stimuli. Superimposed plots of spectra for the *early* window of [kV] produced by speaker N1 are given in Figure 11-3. In this Figure, the [i] vowel is plotted with a solid line. The consonantal spectrum for [ki] shows a sharp spectral peak (2360 Hz) in the *low* frequency region, with no secondary peaks in the *high* frequency region. The consonantal spectrum for [ku] shows a *low* peak at 1236 Hz,

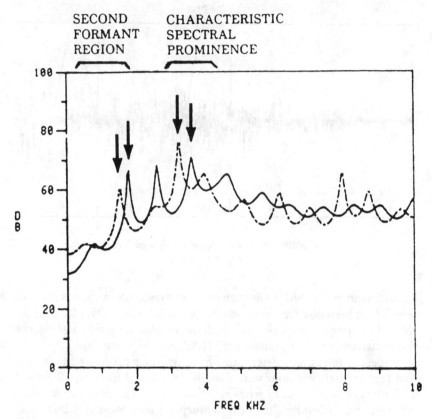

FIGURE 11-2. Spectra of [si] and [su], *late* window. [si] = solid line, [su] = dotted line.

and a secondary *high* frequency peak at 4247 Hz. These peaks are characteristic of front and back [k] allophones in English (Zue, 1976; Stevens & Blumstein, 1978).

Results

Frequency values for spectral peaks were averaged over all repetitions of a given CV or CCV context. These average frequency data are listed in Table 11-1 for normal subjects, Table 11-2 for anterior aphasics, and Table 11-3 for posterior aphasics. The data are arranged by window location (*early* and *late*) and frequency region (*high* and *low*).[1] It will be noted

---

[1]For [kV] syllables, comparisons are made only in the *low* frequency region. This is due to the fact that [k] preceding front vowels does not show secondary peaks in the *high* frequency region (Zue, 1976).

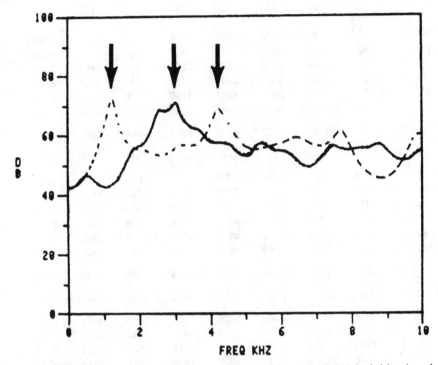

FIGURE 11-3. Superimposed spectra for *early* window of [ki] (solid line) and [ku] (dotted line).

in Table 11-2 that aphasic subjects A4 and A5 did not produce phonemically and phonetically correct tokens of [stV] and [skV].

Turning first to the normal subject data, the principal finding is that in almost every case coarticulatory shifts obtain. The instances in which the values fall in the opposite direction are few (6%), marked in Table 11-1 with asterisks. Similarly, the majority of values (86%) for the aphasic subjects are lower in the context of [u] as compared with [i].

Statistical comparisons indicated that both normal and aphasic subjects showed acoustic correlates of coarticulation. For the CV anticipatory labialization stimuli [sV] and [tV], aphasic subjects' data were statistically indistinguishable from those of the normal subject group, and there were no differences noted as a function of aphasic type. For the anticipatory lingual coarticulation stimuli one statistical difference did emerge: Anterior aphasics produced lower [ki] values than normal and posterior aphasic subjects. However, it was still the case that all groups showed robust [ki/ku] coarticulation. For the consonant cluster stimuli, [stV] and [skV], comparisons between normal and posterior aphasic subjects revealed significant coarticulatory shift for both subject groups. Of the three anterior

TABLE 11-1. Averages of Spectral Peaks, Normal Subjects (n = 6).

Location:	Early				Late			
Frequency:	Low		High		Low		High	
Subject	[si]	[su]	[si]	[su]	[si]	[su]	[si]	[su]
N1	1676	1599	4354	3681	1907	1589	3600	3384
N2	1831	1802	4655	3878	1830	1766	4671	3635
N3	1660	1503	4876	3702	2201	1872	4699	3340
N4	1638	1607	4246	3849	1717	1591	4266	3849
N5	1831	1796	5029	4681	1849	1740	5177	4659
N6	1594*	1614*	5682	4446	1666	1542	4643	4265
x̄	1705	1654	4807	4040	1683		4509	3855
	[sti]	[stu]	[sti]	[stu]	[sti]	[stu]	[sti]	[stu]
N1	1656	1607	4338	3905	1741	1641	4401	3904
N2	1760	1738	4573	3738	1812	1756	4828	3754
N3	1409*	1432*	4553	3467	1623*	1663*	4612	3575
N4	1656	1592	4268	4212	1674	1608	4087	3293
N5	1829	1771	4945	4402	1806	1749	5350	4795
N6	1676	1567	4862	4397	1620*	1665*	5404	4287
x̄	1664	1618	4591	4020	1713	1680	4780	3935
	[ski]	[sku]	[ski]	[sku]	[ski]	[sku]	[ski]	[sku]
N1	2048	1617	4343	3926	2209	1615	4396	3908
N2	1771	1623	4516	3999	1973	1514	4488	3910
N3	1902	1564	4375	3618	1617	1502	4389	3999
N4	1695	1514	4329	4077	1502	1277	4414	3777
N5	1833	1745	4907	4451	2172	1881	4874	4173
N6	2032	1901	4622	4114	1635	1630	4762	3830
x̄	1880	1661	4515	4030	1860	1560	4554	3833
	[ti]	[tu]	[ti]	[tu]	[ti]	[tu]	[ti]	[tu]
N1	1943	1803	3643	3267	2092	1562	3036	2795
N2	1984*	2024*	3649	3234	2070	1916	3906	3693
N3	1937	1784	3387	2929	1938	1517	2985*	3160*
N4	1901	1746	4317	3601	2063	1728	4115	3746
N5	1895	1772	4072	4105	2038	1804	2908*	2909*
N6	2071	1789	3872	2816	2142	1570	3029	2417
x̄	1955	1820	3823	3327	2057	1683	3330	3120
	[ki]	[ku]		[ku]	[ki]	[ku]		[ku]
N1	2942	1295		4517	3090	1297		4261
N2	3120	1428		4459	3125	1475		4448
N3	3045	1155		3960	3015	1044		3869
N4	2708	1342		3555	2741	1223		3742
N5	3061	1604		4095	3126	1670		4410
N6	2888	1099		4067	2806	1161		4178
x̄	2961	1321		4109	2984	1312		4151

TABLE 11-2. Averages of Spectral Peaks, Anterior Aphasic Subjects (n = 5).

Location:	Early				Late			
Frequency:	Low		High		Low		High	
	[si]	[su]	[s i]	[su]	[si]	[su]	[si]	[su]
Subject								
A1	1273	1181	3641	3049	1512*	1605*	3226	2589
A2	2425	1550	4815	3482	2252	1647	4772	3473
A3	1638	1467	3898	3146	1522*	1569*	4171	3136
A4	1692	1644	3416	3048	1703	1534	3688	3175
A5	1681	1530	4249	2849	1605	1469	4159	2254
x̄	1742	1474	4004	3115	1719	1565	4003	2925
	[sti]	[stu]	[s t i]	[stu]	[sti]	[stu]	[sti]	[stu]
A1	1366*	1406*	3412	2640	1331*	1502*	3381	2644
A2	0000	0000	5148	3647	2539	2371	5578	3477
A3	1516*	1554*	4060	3874	2111	2038	3699	3028
A4	—	—	—	—	—	—	—	—
A5	—	—	—	—	—	—	—	—
x̄	1441*	1480*	4027	3387	1994	1970	3219	3050
	[ski]	[sku]	[s k i]	[sku]	[ski]	[sku]	[ski]	[sku]
A1	1202	0000	3182	3026	1813*	1846*	2926	2688
A2	1698*	1724*	4664	3298	1881	1478	4498	3259
A3	1670	1581	3417*	3501*	1602	1505	3500	2981
A4	—	—	—	—	—	—	—	—
A5	—	—	—	—	—	—	—	—
x̄	1523*	1653*	3754	3275	1765	1609	3641	2976
	[ti]	[tu]	[t i]	[tu]	[ti]	[tu]	[ti]	[tu]
A1	1286	1201	2817	2289	0000	1669	2551	2472
A2	2584	1633	4685	2835	1975	1659	2801*	3205*
A3	1862	1605	3438	0000	1807	1645	2650	0000
A4	1660*	1754*	3318	3008	1765	1565	3350	3047
A5	1621	1532	0000	2913	1770	1349	3079	2480
x̄	1803	1545	3564	2761	1829	1577	2886	2801
	[ki]	[ku]		[ku]	[ki]	[ku]		[ku]
A1	2426	1211		4916	2409	1129		0000
A2	2631	1276		4148	1910	1283		4666
A3	2456	1490		3842	2646	1424		4037
A4	1987	1400		0000	2083	1473		3557
A5	2911	1254		3232	2287	1129		3654
x̄	2482	1326		4035	2267	1288		3979

TABLE 11-3. Averages of Spectral Peaks, Posterior Aphasic Subjects (n = 5).

Location:	Early				Late			
Frequency:	Low		High		Low		High	
	[si]	[su]	[s i]	[su]	[si]	[su]	[si]	[su]
Subject								
P1	1997	1949	5441	4012	2063	1818	5326	3693
P2	1788	1488	5585	4481	1744	1523	4647	3799
P3	1608*	1781*	5002	4611	1687	1619	4861	4295
P4	1829*	1841*	4145	3868	1852	1728	4165	3470
P5	1877	1573	3076	2609	1643	1638	2763	2745
x̄	1820	1726	4650	3880	1780	1665	4650	3880
	[sti]	[stu]	[s t i]	[stu]	[sti]	[stu]	[sti]	[stu]
P1	2040	1712	5989	4043	1945	1739	5818	3717
P2	1798	1453	3672*	4006*	1768	1589	5531	4088
P3	1810	1703	4851	4454	1492*	1680*	5137	4868
P4	1879	1811	4200	ˋ3492	1907	1853	4291	3379
P5	1667*	1803*	3536	2736	1909	1747	3565	2788
x̄	1839	1696	4450	3746	1804	1722	4450	3746
	[ski]	[sku]	[s k i]	[sku]	[ski]	[sku]	[ski]	[sku]
P1	1820	1810	6063	3863	1956	1586	3814	3396
P2	1566	1416	0000	3849	1705	1514	5122	3576
P3	1677	1573	5024	3787	1757*	1762*	4952	3489
P4	1688	1598	3667*	3743*	1760	1491	3911	3168
P5	1682*	1747*	3033	2669	2002	1504	3224	2850
x̄	1687	1629	4447	3582	1836	1571	4447	3582
	[ti]	[tu]	[t i]	[tu]	[ti]	[tu]	[ti]	[tu]
P1	1312	1302	0000	3138	2257	1744	3090	2667
P2	1956	1738	3114	3038	1954	1586	2855	2562
P3	1590*	1591*	3196*	3321*	1790	1692	3061	2762
P4	2161	2132	3421	2877	2428	1690	3518	3253
P5	1719	1653	4110	2804	1937	1741	2863	2509
x̄	1748	1683	3460	3036	2073	1691	3460	3036
	[ki]	[ku]		[ku]	[ki]	[ku]		[ku]
P1	2917	1093		4071	3541	1123		4007
P2	2873	1095		3624	3060	1062		3620
P3	3002	1720		4359	3013	1785		3015
P4	2736	1144		3913	2613	1040		3965
P5	3059	1207		4215	2874	1089		4261
x̄	2917	1252		4036	3020	1220		4036

aphasics capable of producing CCV stimuli, subject A2 showed greater than normal degrees of spectral shift in [stV] and [skV], A1 showed roughly normal shift for [stV] but not for [skV], and A3 showed below normal degrees of spectral shift for both [stV] and [skV] stimuli.

In summary, the acoustic data indicate that normal and aphasic subjects show very similar patterns of anticipatory coarticulation for labial and lingual coarticulation in CV syllables. With respect to the CCV stimuli, the results suggest that normal and posterior aphasic subjects produce reliable acoustic correlates of coarticulation for [s] across an intervening stop consonant, while anterior aphasics have more difficulty in producing CCV stimuli, and show appreciable subject-to-subject variation in their responses.

PERCEPTUAL EXPERIMENT

Procedure

The stimuli for the perceptual experiment consisted of a subset of the consonantal segments measured in the acoustic experiment. These stimuli include the [s] portion of [si/su], [sti/stu] and [ski/sku] syllables, the [t] portion of [ti/tu] syllables, and the [k] portion of [ki/ku] syllables. For each syllable types, 5 tokens were randomly selected from the productions of each normal, anterior aphasic and posterior aphasic speaker, yielding a total 760 stimuli. Stimuli were created by sampling tape recordings of subjects' read syllables onto a PDP 11/34 computer and excising the complete aperiodic portion corresponding to the initial [s], [t], and [k] consonants. Digitized audio files were transferred from the computer to a microcomputer adapted for audio playout and subject response monitoring.

Ten students at Brown Univeristy served as paid subjects for the listening experiment. All subjects were native speakers of English, having had no formal training in linguistic theory or phonetics. Subjects were instructed to identify, in a forced choice paradigm, whether the vowels in the test stimuli were either [i] or [u].

Results

Table 11-4 gives listeners' mean correct [i/u] identification scores for productions by normal, anterior and posterior aphasic subjects. Means for the 5 stimulus types are listed at the bottom, and are shown graphically in Figure 11-4. The perceptual scores for productions made by each of the subject groups were found to be significantly above chance. Stimuli produced by normal speakers were correctly identified 84% of the time, anterior aphasics 78%, and posterior aphasics 83%. This indicates that there was sufficient information in the consonant segments taken from CV

TABLE 11-4. Perceptual Results, Item Analysis by Listener.

Speaker:	Normal					Anterior					Posterior				
	[s]	[st]	[sk]	[t]	[k]	[s]	[st]	[sk]	[t]	[k]	[s]	[st]	[sk]	[t]	[k]
Listener:															
KM	76	68	70	97	98	60	72	70	69	93	81	65	79	92	100
TD	73	63	71	93	95	73	83	72	75	95	74	62	77	93	99
AP	79	73	81	90	98	76	73	72	73	97	68	68	90	81	92
JK	81	63	73	95	99	56	65	63	69	95	66	57	77	89	97
BD	68	66	72	92	100	64	53	73	69	89	65	61	69	87	97
JL	88	76	80	96	99	79	90	67	84	94	92	77	90	96	96
SF	92	78	79	93	99	85	85	70	75	96	79	69	86	98	100
LD	89	78	84	95	100	91	82	73	77	95	92	72	80	97	98
DO	76	66	79	88	94	80	80	68	78	95	73	64	76	88	94
JB	91	75	77	96	100	84	77	72	82	99	80	74	85	95	99
x	81	71	77	94	98	75	76	70	75	95	77	67	81	91	97
SD	8	6	5	3	2	11	11	3	5	3	10	6	7	5	3

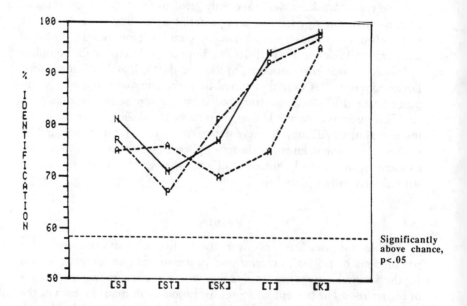

FIGURE 11-4. Mean correct identification scores for productions by normal (N), anterior (A), and posterior (P) aphasic subjects.

and CCV productions by normal and aphasic speakers to allow listeners to identify the subsequent vowel.

Figure 11-4 shows that identification varies as a function of *group* and *stimulus* type. Overall, productions by anterior aphasic speakers were identified with lower degrees of accuracy than were stimuli produced by normal and posterior aphasic subjects. The one exception was for [stV] stimuli, for which anterior aphasics' productions showed greater identification scores than normal subjects' productions.[2] In contrast, the only case in which identification values for normal and posterior aphasic productons differed was in [skV] stimuli, with posterior aphasic productions having higher values than those of normal subjects.

If the data are considered by *stimulus* type, i.e., collapsing across *groups* [kV] stimuli show the greatest correct identification (97%), followed by [tV] (92%), [skV] (81%), [sV] (77%), and [stV] (67%). Statistical comparisons showed overall differences between each stimulus type, with the exception of [s]/[sk]. That is, the stimuli may be ranked from highest to lowest correct identification as follows:

$$[kV] > [tV] > [sV] > [stV]$$
$$[skV]$$

CORRELATION BETWEEN ACOUSTIC AND PERCEPTUAL DATA

The acoustic and perceptual results both show that normal and aphasic subjects produce quantifiable coarticulatory shifts. In addition, if the data are considered by *stimulus* type, there is good general agreement between the acoustic and the perceptual data. For example, the stimuli with the greatest amount of perceptual identification, [kV], showed the greatest degree of coarticulatory shift, while the stimuli showing the lowest perceptual scores, [stV], showed the least amount of spectral shift. However, for [tV] and [skV] stimuli, the acoustic data showed greater coarticulatory shift for [skV] than for [tV], while the perceptual data showed the opposite pattern, i.e., 92% identification for [tV] and 81% identification for [skV]. In addition, *group* differences emerged in the perceptual but not in the acoustic data.

As a further means of comparing the acoustic and perceptual data, an analysis was conducted in order to determine which of the four spectral measures used in the acoustic analysis (*early-low, early-high, late-low,*

---

[2]It must be recalled that there were only 3 anterior aphasics who could produce CCV stimuli. Thus, the "higher than normal" identification scores for anterior aphasics' [stV] stimuli may not constitute a *group* effect. The elevated [stV] mean for the anterior aphasics is mainly due to productions by subject A2, which showed 88% correct identification.

late-high) best predicts listeners' perceptual responses. A series of sample Pearson correlation coefficients was calculated for the perceptual and acoustic parameters. These data indicated that *late-low* acoustic measures best predict the normal-posterior aphasic group data. In contrast, the anterior subject data showed that *early-high* (r = .81) and *early/low* (r = .56) were the most strongly correlated variables, both being significant at p < .05.

GENERAL DISCUSSION

The main finding of both the acoustic and perceptual experiments is that aphasic subjects' CV and CCV productions show clear evidence of anticipatory coarticulation. This first of all demonstrates that both anterior and posterior aphasic subjects retain coarticulatory planning processes for CV and CCV syllable-sized units. This finding supports the claim by Buckingham (1981), based on observations of preposturing behavior, that although anterior aphasic subjects may evidence sequencing impairments, they appear to anticipate lip-rounding in speech planning.

The current data also show that the actual *implementation* ("phasing," "transitionalizing") of planned coarticulatory gestures is intact in posterior aphasia, and is only partially affected in anterior aphasia. These data are in agreement with the findings of Itoh et al. (1979), who conducted a fibroscopic investigation of nasalization in the speech of a 51-year-old anterior aphasic subject. Although slight disturbances in the synchronization of time schedules for velar lowering were noted, the authors concluded that anticipatory coarticulation for nasalization was for the most part intact in this subject's speech.

With respect to neurolinguistic models of speech production, the data from these two experiments suggest that coarticulatory information is likely encoded in the most basic elements of the speech production process. In other words, the data do not support a speech production model in which there are separable levels or "modules" of processing in which speech represented is distinct segments (or phonemes) devoid of coarticulatory information. Rather, the present findings mitigate against theories which propose local modules for "motor preprogramming" in specific cortical regions such as Broca's area (e.g., Luria, 1966; Darley, Aronson, & Brown, 1975; Mlcoch & Noll, 1980), and instead appear to be better explained by "global" models that propose that the participation of several neural structures is involved in the processing of speech production (e.g., Brown, 1975; Requin, 1980). Future work making use of more detailed measurements will hopefully shed light on these issues.

Although the acoustic and perceptual data show reliable coarticulation in the speech of normal and aphasic subjects, it was also observed that the perceptual scores for the anterior aphasic stimuli were lower than those for the normal subject stimuli. These data conform with the general clinical picture of anterior aphasics exhibiting nonfluent, poorly articulated speech, and posterior aphasics exhibiting fluent, well-articulated speech. These findings also support the "phonetic versus phonemic" processing distinction felt to characterize the speech production of anterior versus posterior aphasics (Blumstein, 1981; 1986; Ryalls, 1986). The fact that posterior aphasics pattern very similarly to normal subjects suggests that the "subtle phonetic deficit" noted to exist in posterior aphasics' speech does not extend to anticipatory coarticulation processes.

The finding that the overall perceptual scores for the anterior aphasic productions were lower than those of the normal subjects does allow for the possibility that anterior aphasic subjects demonstrate a slight delay (Zeigler & von Cramon, 1985, 1986, 1986b) or deficiency (Tuller & Story, 1986) in anticipatory coarticulation. However, a close inspection of the present data mitigates against these hypotheses. Although the present experiments were not designed to explore in detail the time course of coarticulation, the acoustic data do shed some light on the timing question. It was found that for normal and anterior aphasic subjects there were no significant differences in the amount of coarticulatory shift found in *early* vs. *late* portions of fricatives, and there was statistically significant shift present in the *early* region (i.e., the release) of [t] and [k] stop consonants. These findings are not consistent with the notion of a "delay" of labialization in anterior subjects' speech, but instead suggest that anterior aphasic subjects initiate coarticulatory gestures at least as early as normal as subjects.[3]

In addition, it is important to note that the decrements in anterior aphasics' productions are not "across the board," but differ with stimulus type. That is, [kV] stimuli show no differences between anterior aphasics and normal subjects, [tV] stimuli show large differences, [sV] and [skV] show small but reliable differences, and [stV] stimuli fall in the opposite direction (with anterior aphasics showing a normal or greater-than-normal degree of coarticulation). The view that anterior aphasics have overall deficits or delays in coarticulation is not sufficient to describe this pattern of results. Rather, it appears that taking stimulus-specific motor and timing information into account may provide more suitable explanations for anterior aphasics' deficits. Let us consider the data by stimulus type. The finding that anterior aphasics show "normal" patterns of coarticulation for the velar stimuli, [kV], demonstrates that these subjects are able to

---

[3]Although it must be recalled that the *early* window for fricatives in this study was placed not at the onset of frication, but at a location 70 ms prior to the end of frication. It thus remains a possibility that normal versus aphasic differences might be found at an earlier point in the frication.

select the correct /k/ allophone and place their articulators in an appropriate position for production. This finding agrees with the hypothesis by Shinn and Blumstein (1983) that anterior aphasic subjects show a relatively preserved ability to reach the appropriate place of articulation for stop consonants. In contrast, anterior aphasics have documented difficulties with speech production processes requiring the coordination of two or more independent articulators in the production of the phonetic dimensions of voicing and nasality as well as in laryngeal control (Blumstein et al., 1977/1980; Itoh et al., 1979/1980/1982; Freeman et al., 1978; Shewan et al., 1982; Tuller, 1984; Gandour & Dardarananda, 1984). This dichotomy between "global" articulatory impairments and impairments that affect the coordination of two (or more) independent articulators would explain why anterior aphasics are able to perform within normal limits in velar coarticulation, which requires coordination of a single articulator (the tongue), but not in anticipatory labilization, which requires simultaneous programming of the tongue and lips.

The poor identification of anterior aphasics' [tV] stimuli might involve a greater relative difficulty in control of fine movements of the tongue blade (a theory proposed by Shinn & Blumstein, 1983). This, in turn, might be related to the fact that stops require relatively rapid gestues, e.g., as compared with fricatives. For example, in [t] production, the tongue blade moves rapidly from the alveolar ridge, whereas [s] is produced by maintaining a constriction between the tongue blade and the alveolar ridge for a much longer period of time. These factors would provide an explanation for anterior aphasics' [tV] productions showing greater impairments than their [sV] productions. An explanation in terms of articulatory difficulty might also explain why [skV] stimuli showed coarticulatory deficiencies, while the perceptual scores for [stV] stimuli were equal to or better than normal subjects' productions. The consonants in [stV] stimuli share the alveolar place of articulation, and require only a slight raising of the tongue to move from a fricative to a stop. In contrast, for [skV] production it is necessary to coordinate two separate parts of the same articulator, i.e., the tongue blade and body, over both front and back regions of the mouth. Thus, it may be reasoned that [skV] stimuli are more "difficult" to articulate than [stV] stimuli. On this view, postulated deficits for anterior aphasics involving "two independent articulators" might also affect articulation involving two different regions of the same articulator (e.g., tongue blade and body). Again, these theories are speculative and will require further study before conclusions can be drawn.

Let us next consider the relation between the acoustic and perceptual data. The current series of experiments showed reasonably good agreement between acoustic and perceptual results, however a number of differences were noted: For [tV] and [skV] stimuli, the acoustic data showed greater coarticulatory shift for [skV] than for [tV], while the perceptual data showed the opposite pattern. In addition, there were no *group* differences observed in the acoustic data, whereas in the perceptual data productions by anterior aphasics received lower overall identification scores. There are several possible explanations for these differences. First, it is possible that LPC made errors for the stimuli analyzed. LPC analysis assumes an all-pole model of speech production, and may therefore make substantial errors when used to analyze fricatives and stop consonants (stimuli that contain zeros, as well as poles). It would be useful to attempt to replicate the present results (as well as the results of other LPC studies, e.g., Ziegler & von Cramon, 1985, 1986a, 1986b; Tuller & Story, 1986) using more advanced methods of LPC analysis which are based on a pole-zero representation, such as those being developed by Atal and Schroeder (1978). Nevertheless, the fact that there were areas of good agreement between the perceptual and acoustic data, e.g., with respect to the magnitude of coarticulation for each stimulus type, makes it seem unlikely that overall LPC errors explain the pattern of results. A more likely explanation may be that the spectral parameters measured from the LPC plots, i.e., second formant and CSP peaks, are not the only information used by listeners in their perceptual judgments. Instead, it seems reasonable to assume that listeners make use of a complex series of spectral cues for the determination of coarticulatory vowel information in consonantal portions of the waveform. This may include more "global" properties of the waveform, such as overall spectral shape, or concentrations of energy in relatively wide bandwidth portions of the spectrum.

The results of the correlation analyses showed that specific peaks in different areas of the waveform are more predictive of perceptual responses than are other peaks. For example, *late-low* (i.e., second formant peaks sampled 20 ms prior to the end of the consonantal portion of the waveform) best predict the perceptual findings for normal and posterior aphasic subjects' productions. These data replicate the findings of earlier research with normal subjects (Soli, 1981; Sereno et al., 1987). The findings that a different set of acoustic measures predicted the perceptual data for anterior aphasics' productions, i.e., *early-high* and (to a lesser extent) *early-low* peaks, suggest that the early portions of anterior aphasics' stimuli contain relatively more stable coarticulatory cues than are found in the spectra of normal and posterior aphasic subjects' productions. Additional research will be needed in order to determine the exact nature of the perceptually salient spectral cues for the perception of coarticulation.

REFERENCES

Alajuounine, T., Ombredane, A., & Durand, M. (1939). *Le syndrome de désintegraton phonétique dans l' aphasie.* Paris: Masson et Cie.

Atal, B.S., & Schroeder, M.R. (1978). Linear prediction analysis of speech based on a pole-zero representation. *Journal of the Acoustical Society of America, 64,* 1310–1318.

Blumstein, S.E. (1973). *A phonological investigation of aphasic speech*. The Hague: Mouton.

Blumstein, S.E. (1981). Phonological aspects of aphasia. In M.T. Sarno (Ed.), *Acquired aphasia*. New York: Academic Press.

Blumstein, S.E. (1986). Neurolinguistics: An overview of language-brain relations in aphasia. In F. Newmeyer (Ed.), *Linguistics: The Cambridge survey*. Cambridge University Press.

Blumstein, S.E., Cooper, W.E., Zurif, E.B. & Carmazza, A. (1977). The perception and production of voice-onset time in aphasia. *Neuropsychologia, 15*, 371–383.

Blumstein, S.E., & Stevens, K.N. (1979). Acoustic invariance in speech production: Evidence for measurements of the spectral characteristics of stop consonants. *Journal of the Acoustical Society of America, 66*, 1001–1017.

Blumstein, S.E., Cooper, W.E., Goodglass, H., Statlender, S., & Gottlieb, J. (1980). Production deficits in aphasia: A voice onset time analysis. *Brain and Language, 9*, 153–170.

Brown, J.W. (1975). On the neural organization of language: Thalamic and cortical relations. *Brain and Language 2*, 18–30.

Buckingham, H.W. (1981). Explanations for the concept of apraxia of speech. In M. Sarno, (Ed.), *Acquired aphasia*. New York: Academic Press.

Darley, F.L., Aronson, A.E., & Brown, J.R. (1975). *Motor speech disorders*. Philadelphia: Saunders.

Fant, G. (1973). Stops in CV syllables. In G. Fant (Ed.), *Speech sounds and features*. Cambridge: MIT Press.

Freeman, F.J., Sands, E.S., & Harris, K.S. (1978). Temporal coordination of phonation and articulation in a case of verbal apraxia: A voice onset time study. *Brain and Language, 6*, 106–111.

Gandour, J. & Dardarananda, R. (1984). Voice onset in aphasia: Thai, II. Production. *Brain and Language, 23*, 177–205.

Goodglass, H., & Kaplan, E. (1983). *The assessment of aphasia and related disorders*. Philadelphia: Lea and Febinger.

Halle, M., Hughes, G. & Radley, J.P.A. (1957). Acoustic perception of stop consonants. *Journal of the Acoustical Society of America, 29*, 107–116.

Itoh, M., Sasanuma, S., & Ushijima, T. (1979). Velar movements during speech in a patient with apraxia of speech. *Brain and Language, 7*, 227–239.

Itoh, M., Sasanuma, S., Hirose, H., Yoshioka, H., & Ushijima, T. (1980). Abnormal articulatory dynamics in a patient with apraxia of speech: X-ray microbeam observation. *Brain and Language, 11*, 66–75.

Itoh, M., Sasanuma, S., Tatsumi, I., Murakami, S., Fukusato, Y., & Suzuki, T. (1982). Voice onset time characteristics in apraxia of speech. *Brain and Language, 17*, 193–210.

Katz, W. (1987). *An acoustic and perceptual investigation of anticipatory coarticulation in aphasia*. (Unpublished Ph.D. dissertation, Brown University).

LaRiviere, C., Winitz, H., Herriman, E. (1975a). Vocalic transitions in the perception of voiceless initial stops. *Journal of the Acoustical Society of America, 57*, 470–475.

LaRiviere, C., Winitz, H., & Herriman, E. (1975b). The distribution of perceptual cues in English prevocalic fricatives. *Journal of Speech and Hearing Research, 18*, 613–622.

Lieberman, P., & Sereno, J. (1986). Developmental aspects of the production of velar stop consonants. *Journal of the Acoustical Society of America (Suppl. 1)*, 79, s54.

Lubker, J.F., & Gay, T. (1982). Anticipatory labial coarticulation: Experimental, biological, and linguistic variables. *Journal of the Acoustical Society of America*, 17(2), 437–447.

Luria, A.R. (1966). *Higher cortical functions in man.* New York: Basic Books.

Mertus, J. (1980). *WAVED Waveform editing manual*, Brown University Department of Linguistics.

Mlcoch, A.G., & Noll, J.D. (1980). Speech production models as related to the concept of apraxia of speech. In N.J. Lass (Ed), *Speech and language: Advances in basic research and practice (Vol. 4)*, pp. 201–239.

Ohde, R.N., & Sharf, D.J. (1977). Order effect of acoustic segments of VC and CV syllables on stop and vowel identification. *Journal of Speech and Hearing Research*, 20, 543–554.

Ohde, R.N., & Sharf, D.J. (1981). Physiological, acoustic, and perceptual aspects of coarticulation: Implications for the remediation of articulatory disorders. In N.J. Lass (Ed.), *Speech and language: Advances in basic research (Vol. 5)*. New York: Academic Press.

Ohman, S.E.G. (1966). Coarticulation in VCV utterances: Spectrographic measurements. *Journal of the Acoustical Society of America*, 39, 151–168.

Peterson, G.E., & Lehiste, I. (1960). Duration of syllabic nuclei in English. *Journal of the Acoustical Society of America*, 32, 693–703.

Potter, R.K., Kopp, G.A., & Green, H.C. (1947). *Visible speech.* New York: Van Nostrand.

Rabiner, L.R., & Schafter, J. (1979). *Digital processing of speech.* New York: McGraw-Hill.

Requin, J. (1980). Towards a psychobiology of preparation for action. In G.E. Stelmach & J. Requin (Eds.), *Tutorials in motor behavior.* Amsterdam: North-Holland.

Ryalls, J.H. (1982). Intonation in Broca's aphasia. *Neuropsychologia*, 20, 355–360.

Ryalls, J.H. (1984). Some acoustic aspects of fundamental frequency of CVC utterances in aphasia. *Phonetica*, 41, 103–111.

Ryalls, J.H. (1986). An acoustic study of vowel production in aphasia. *Brain and Language*, 29, 48–67.

Sands, E.S., Freeman, F.J., & Harris, K.S. (1978). Progressive changes in articulatory patterns in verbal apraxia: A longitudinal case study. *Brain and Language*, 6, 97–105.

Schatz, D. (1954). The role of context in the perception of stops. *Language*, 30, 47–56.

Sereno, J.A., Baum, S.R., Marean, G.C., & Lieberman, P. (1987). Acoustic analyses and perceptual data on anticipatory labial coarticulation in adults and children. *Journal of the Acoustical Society of America*, 81, 512–519.

Shankweiler, D. & Harris, K.S. (1966). An experimental approach to the problem of articulation in aphasia. *Cortex*, 2, 277–292.

Shewan, C., Leeper, H., & Booth (1984). An analysis of voice onset time (VOT) in aphasic and normal subjects. In Rosensbek, J., McNeil, M.R., & Aronson, A.E., (Eds.), *Apraxia of Speech.* San Diego, CA: College-Hill Press.

Shinn, P., & Blumstein, S.B. (1983). Phonetic disintegration in aphasia: Acoustic analysis of spectral characteristics for place of articulation. *Brain and Language*, 20, 90–114.

Soli, S. (1981). Second formants in fricatives: Acoustic consequences of fricative-vowel coarticulation. *Journal of the Acoustical Society of America*, 70, 976–984.

Stevens, K.N., & Blumstein, S.E. (1978). Invariant cues for place of articulation in stop consonants. *Journal of the Acoustical Society of America*, 64, 1358–1368.

Tikofsky, R. (1965). *Phonetic characteristics of dysarthria*. Ann Arbor: Office of Research Administration. The University of Michigan.

Tuller, B. (1984). On categorizing aphasic speech errors. *Neuropsychologia*, 22(5), 547–557.

Tuller, B., & Story, R.S. (1986). Co-articulation in aphasic speech. *Journal of the Acoustical Society of America (Suppl. 1)*, 80, MM17.

Turnbaugh, K.R., Hoffman, P.R., & Daniloff, R.G. (1985). Stop-vowel coarticulation in a 3-year-old, 5-year-old, and adult speakers. *Journal of the Acoustical Society of America*, 77, 1256–1257.

Winitz, H., Scheib, M.E., & Reeds, J.A. (1972). Identification of stops and vowels for the burst portion of /p,t,k/ isolated from conversational speech. *Journal of the Acoustical Society of America*, 51, 1309–1317.

Yeni-Komshian, G., & Soli, S. (1981). Recognition of vowels from information in fricatives: Perceptual evidence of fricative-vowel coarticulation. *Journal of the Acoustical Society of America*, 70, 966–975.

Ziegler, W., & von Cramon, D. (1985). Anticipatory coarticulation in a patient with apraxia of speech. *Brain and Language*, 26, 117–130.

Ziegler, W., & von Cramon, D. (1986a). Disturbed coarticulation in apraxia of speech: Acoustic evidence. *Brain and Language*, 29, 34–47.

Ziegler, W., & von Cramon, D. (1986b). Timing deficits in apraxia of speech. *European Archives of Psychiatric and Neurological Science*, 236, 44–49.

Zue, V. (1976). *Acoustic characteristics of stop consonants: A controlled study* (Unpublished Ph.D. dissertation, MIT).

Anticipatory Coarticulation in Aphasia

Betty Tuller
Robin Seider Story

A standard view of speech production is that it entails two relatively independent terminal stages—one in which speech segments (such as consonants and vowels) are selected and sequenced, and a second stage in which segments are executed by the speech motor system (e.g., Kent, 1976). The most compelling evidence for these two independent stages is the production of speech errors in which two segments exchange positions but are nevertheless produced correctly in their new context (MacKay, 1970). This has been interpreted as evidence that the movements for production of segments are planned after the order of segments has been assigned (MacNeilage, 1980).

This two-stage view also characterizes descriptions of aphasic speech. Traditional clinical descriptions of aphasia consider most errors in speech produced by posterior, fluent (Wernicke's) aphasics to originate at the level of phonemic or phonological selection and ordering. So-called "phonetic" errors, arising at the level of speech-motor control, are thought to be more typical of anterior, nonfluent (Broca's) aphasics (Alajouanine, Ombredane, & Durand, 1939: Luria, 1966; Shankweiler & Harris, 1966). Although work in the last decade has in general supported this dichotomy, a number of studies have shown that some apparently phonemic errors may in fact be phonetically-based distortions.[1] In the following, we will briefly consider such evidence from physiological studies, phonetic transcriptions, and acoustic analyses.

---

[1]Heeding Buckingham's (1981) warning that the phonemic and phonetic distinction properly refers to a linguistic level of description, not a processing level, we will in this chapter use the terms *premotoric* and *motoric* (cf. MacNeilage, Hutchinson, & Lasater, 1981).

Physiological study is by far the least common but most direct method used in investigations of speech produced by aphasics. Nevertheless, the studies that have been performed suggest strongly that some apparently premotoric errors may in fact be motorically based, at least in nonfluent aphasia. For example, Shankweiler, Harris, and Taylor (1968) studied electromyographic patterns of lip and tongue muscles during speech produced by two nonfluent aphasic subjects with apraxia of speech. Both subjects showed highly variable timing and duration of muscle activity patterns, in comparison with normal subjects.

Itoh and his colleages in Japan have provided most of the existing empirical analyses of articulator movements produced by aphasic speakers (e.g., Itoh, Sasanuma, & Ushijima, 1979; Itoh, et al., 1980). For example, they report that a nonfluent aphasic speaker with apraxia of speech shows abnormal temporal coordination of velar and tongue movements for production of nasal consonants. On occasion, the relative timing of lingual and velar movements was sufficiently disrupted to result in a sound change transcribed as a "phonemic" error.

A second, more indirect source of evidence for abnormal speech-motor patterning in aphasia is phonetic transcription of speech. Using this technique, Blumstein (1973) explored whether Broca's aphasics, Wernicke's aphasics, and conduction aphasics tend to substitute unmarked consonants for marked ones. Unmarked consonants (such as the alveolar consonant /t/) usually occur earlier in children's speech and are more common across the world's languages than are marked sounds (such as the palatal consonant /č/). Unmarked sounds are therefore thought to be easier to produce. If aphasic errors are not solely of linguistic origin, but also involve a motoric component, one might expect Broca's aphasics, whose productions are often described as "distorted" or "incoordinated," to substitute unmarked sounds for marked ones. This was in fact the pattern Blumstein (1973) observed. More surprising, however, was that the same substitution pattern was observed for all three aphasic groups (see also Marquardt, Rinehart, & Peterson, 1979; MacNeilage, Hutchinson & Lasater, 1981).

A third source of support for the idea that motoric processes may underlie apparently premotoric errors, particularly in Broca's aphasia, is provided by studies that examine the acoustic speech signal as a window into the origin of speech production errors. For example, one commonly measured aspect of aphasic speech is voice-onset time (VOT). VOT is defined as the time between the release of supraglottal occlusion for a stop consonant and the onset of glottal pulsing or voicing. Thus, it is an acoustic indication of the time between two articulatory events. In the production of English voiced stop consonants in syllable-initial position, glottal pulsing begins anywhere from approximately 100 ms before, to 20 ms after, release of the stop consonant. In syllable-initial, voiceless stop consonants, glottal pulsing begins approximately 40 to 150 ms after stop consonant release (Lisker & Abramson, 1967).

The patterning of VOT across voiced and voiceless stop consonants produced by aphasic speakers is by now fairly well-documented (e.g. Blumstein et al., 1977, 1980; Freeman, Sands, & Harris, 1978; Hoit-Dalgaard, Murry, & Koop, 1983; Shewan, Leeper, & Booth, 1984; Tuller, 1984). By and large, the results across studies are remarkably stable. Broca's aphasics, Wernicke's aphasics, and conduction aphasics all produce instances of phonetic-motoric errors (defined as consonants produced with VOTs intermediate between those typical of normal voiced and voiceless consonants) as well as instances of phonemic-premotoric errors (defined by productions of consonants with VOT values within the normal range of the consonant opposite in voicing to the one required). In general, Broca's aphasics tend to make more motoric errors than do Wernicke's or conduction aphasics. Many of these objectively motoric errors could be transcribed as phonemic substitutions. Moreover, only the Broca's aphasics tended to produce relatively more motoric errors than premotoric errors. Similar motoric deficits have been reported for aphasic speakers of Japanese (Itoh et al., 1980) and Thai (Gandour & Dardarananda, 1984).

In summary, physiological, linguistic, and acoustic studies all support the hypothesis that both Broca's and Wernicke's aphasics show some form of articulatory difficulty regardless of the associated language disturbance. Although the articulatory disruptions are evident across aphasia types, they are as a rule more severe in Broca's aphasia. Nevertheless, the results do little toward explaining why speech of Broca's aphasics and Wernicke's aphasics is perceptually so different. This may be in part because theoretical conclusions have been based on productions that are perceived as errors. This necessarily restricts the available data base and, because of the variability in aphasic speaker's output, makes comparisons across experiments, across speakers, or even across experimental sessions, extremely difficult.

There is accumulating evidence that abnormal articulatory patterns also occur during perceptually correct tokens of aphasic speech. In Blumstein et al. (1977; 1980) when Broca's aphasics produced "correct" VOT values for the required consonant, the overall VOT distribution was still very different from the normal pattern, suggesting a "pervasive phonetic disorder" (Blumstein et al., 1980). Wernicke's "correct" productions of voiced stop consonants tended to have a longer voicing lead, and more prevoicing, than produced by normal subjects. Thus, analysis of perceptually correct speech output might allow a controlled study of articulatory patterns in aphasia in which variability can be assessed across multiple tokens of a word produced by a single aphasic speaker as well as for the same word set across speakers.

A second and related explanation for why objective measures have yielded surprisingly similar descriptions of Broca's and Wernicke's aphasia may be the emphasis of previous research on cues for segmental distinctions, particularly those, like VOT, with an absolute temporal criterion. In contrast to VOT, most other acoustic temporal cues for segmental distinctions cannot be defined according to an absolute temporal boundary. For example, the voicing distinction for stop consonants in medial position is cued in part by the duration of silence preceding the consonant release. However, the duration of silence necessary to specify that the medial stop consonant is voiceless, and not voiced, decreases as speaking rate increases (Port, 1979). Nonfluent aphasics tend to produce longer segments, words and sentences than do normal speakers, and with higher than normal variability (e.g., Ryalls, 1981; Collins et al., 1983; Kent & Rosenbek, 1983; Williams & Seaver, 1986). It is perhaps not surprising, then, that investigations of aphasic speech that measured a distinction based on relative time have not been as stable as those that measured an absolute temporal distinction. For example, Duffy & Gawle (1984) reported that aphasic speakers use vowel duration as a cue to final consonant voicing, whereas Tuller (1984) often observed this cue to be disrupted.

A third shortcoming of previous work is the equating of motoric events with the production of individual segments. Historically, the two-stage model of speech production assumes that planned segments are discrete, static and context-free, whereas uttered segments are overlapped, dynamic, and context-sensitive (e.g. Hockett, 1955; MacNeilage & Ladefoged, 1976). Thus, it is extremely difficult, if not impossible, to identify the canonical units of phonology in either articulatory gestures or the acoustic signal. The rules for such "coarticulation" of segments remains a matter of some controversy, as does the nature of the segments themselves. Nevertheless, it is by now well-established that coarticulation is not to be viewed as unwanted articulatory noise that serves only to obscure the identity of segments. Rather, the acoustic consequences of coarticulated speech are themselves extremely informative for the listener (cf. Elman & McClelland, 1983). Abnormal coarticulatory patterns have been associated with extreme perceptual distortions, as in speech of the profoundly deaf (McGarr & Harris, 1983; McGarr, Kobayashi, & Honda, 1984).

Uncovering the basis for normal coarticulatory patterns has been a major thrust of speech production research. Yet surprisingly little is known concerning the preservation or disruption of coarticulation in aphasic speakers. This information would be particularly useful given the evidence reviewed above that patients with Broca's aphasia, or speech apraxia, have difficulty coordinating the articulatory movements for a single speech sound. That articulation across segments is also disrupted has been suggested by Ziegler and von Cramon (1985, 1986a, 1986b). First, those authors reported a disturbed pattern of anticipatory coarticulation in one nonfluent aphasic speaker with speech apraxia, whether anticipation was measured acoustically or perceptually. Next, the authors showed the same disrupted acoustic pattern for 6 subjects with apraxia of speech. Unfortunately, the 6 apraxic subjects included 2 subjects with Broca's aphasia,

2 subjects with Wernicke's aphasia, 1 subject with Conduction aphasia, and 1 subject whose aphasia was not classifiable. Despite this heterogeneity, only grouped data were analyzed, perhaps because each subject produced only two tokens of each stimulus word.

Itoh et al. (1979) also examined anticipatory velar lowering for production of a nasal consonant for a single apraxic speaker. They note that in correct productions, the apraxic patient lowered his velum at the appropriate relative time within the syllable despite extremely variable segment durations. In one instance, however, velar lowering began much earlier than normal. This hint that apraxic speakers may show an increased extent of anticipatory coarticulation is contrary to the data of Ziegler and von Cramon (1986a, 1986b) but supported by those of Katz (this volume) and by informal observations of these patients' "preposturing" behavior (Buckingham, 1981). In a second instance reported by Itoh et al. (1979), velar lowering and tongue-tip movements were mistimed, resulting in the perceived substitution of [d] for [n]. However, it is unclear whether the mistiming entailed the tongue tip raising too early, or the velum lowering too late. Thus, the question remains open of whether aphasia or apraxia of speech disrupts the temporal extent of coarticulatory gestures.

The present study expands on this issue in two ways. First, we explore anticipatory coarticulatory patterns in speech of Wernicke's and Broca's aphasics, with and without speech apraxia and agrammatism, in order to explore whether the pattern of results found with speech apraxia is common across different types of aphasia. Second, the procedures elicit a large enough set of utterances so that subjects can be examined individually. The coarticulatory phenomenon chosen for study is the well-documented anticipation of lip rounding that occurs before rounded vowels such as /u/ and the consequent lowering of the spectra of a prevocalic fricative (e.g. Hughes & Halle, 1956; Jassem, 1964; Soli, 1981). In particular, Soli (1981) observed that the spectral peaks in alveolar fricatives, also used in the present study, are associated with vocal tract resonances that clearly determine the second formant of a following high vowel (/i/ or /u/). In other words, the spectral peaks in alveolar fricatives are a consistent product of anticipatory vowel coarticulation. The question addressed here is whether the normal course of anticipatory vowel coarticulation is disrupted in Broca's or Wernicke's aphasia.

METHOD

Subjects

The subjects in this study included 5 fluent (Wernicke's) aphasics (referred to hereafter as FL1 through FL5), 5 nonfluent (Broca's) aphasics (referred to as NF1 through NF5), and 5 control speakers (C1 through

C5). The diagnostic category of each patient was determined by performance on the Boston Diagnostic Aphasia Examination (BDAE; Goodglass & Kaplan, 1972) and other neurological and neuropsychological tests. Only those aphasics on whom there was a clinical consensus were included.

The fluent aphasics were articulatorily agile and used phrases of normal length. However, their speech often made no sense. All of the nonfluent aphasics spoke hesitantly, with long pauses between words, that is, in an "effortful" manner. Three of the nonfluent aphasics would be characterized as having agrammatic output (NFl, NF2, and NF5) and three as having apraxia of speech (NF3, NF4, and NF5). Those subjects called agrammatic, in addition to meeting the BDAE criteria for Broca's aphasia, produced speech characterized by the omission of grammatical morphemes, loss of verb-subject agreement, and failure to use proper inflections. The presence of speech apraxia was assessed using a list of 35 monosyllabic and polysyllabic words and sentences selected from a larger list provided by Darley, Aronson, and Brown (1975). A speaker was diagnosed as "apraxic" if production of the list contained numerous but inconsistent phonetic errors of various types that increased with sentence length, as well as attempts at self-correction. The errors were judged by a linguist who had no information concerning the individual patients.

In all cases, etiology was vascular and involved only the left hemisphere. No tumor or trauma cases were included. All of the subjects were right-handed premorbidly. The 5 right-handed control subjects were selected to span the age range of the aphasic subjects. Supplementary information concerning the aphasic subjects is presented in Table 12-1.

Stimuli

The subjects were required to produce 16 two-word sequences of which the following subset of 8 sequences comprises the corpus for the present experiment.

pea soup	new seat
these soups	whose seat
we seek	new suit
these seats	whose suit

Notice that the vowels include all four combinations of /i/ and /u/. Half the word pairs contain an intervocalic, word-final /z/ and word-initial /s/ (e.g., *these soups*) and half the word pairs contain only the word-initial /s/ (e.g., *pea soup*).

Procedure

Each word pair was printed in large block letters on an index card and presented to the subject in random order. On presentation of the card, subjects were required to read the word pair aloud at least twice. If the

TABLE 12-1. Descriptive Data for Aphasic Subjects

Speaker Type	Age	Sex	Years of Schooling	Year of Onset	Auditory* Comprehension	Hemiplegia
Fluent						
FL1	57	F	16	1972	+.7	No
FL2	67	F	16	1969	−.3	No
FL3	49	M	16	1977	+.06	No
FL4	55	M	10	1976	−.12	No
FL5	43	M	14	1972	−.6	No
Nonfluent						
NF1[†]	61	F	16	1979	+.2	No
NF2[†]	66	M	12	1980	.0	Yes
NF3[‡]	67	M	4	1979	+.7	Yes
NF4[‡]	69	M	20	1980	+1.0	Yes
NF5[†‡]	52	M	8	1974	+1.0	Yes

*Mean of the four auditory comprehension subtests of the Boston Diagnostic Aphasia Examination (Goodglass & Kaplan, 1972)
[†]Agrammatism
[‡]Speech apraxia

subject was unable to read the card easily, the experimenter would conceal his or her mouth with an index card and pronounce the word pair for the subject to repeat. The randomized list of sequences was presented a minimum of 8 times so that each subject attempted to produce at least 16 tokens of each word pair. Subject responses were recorded onto a high-quality tape recorder for later analysis. Each subject was tested individually in a sound-insulated room.

Data Analysis

Broad phonemic transcriptions of all utterances were made by a linguist who was unfamiliar with the stimulus set and the speakers. Target segments transcribed as a different phoneme from that required were excluded from further analysis. In addition, two members of the University's secretarial staff were asked to identify the produced sequences. Only word pairs that both listeners correctly identified were included in the spectral analysis. Across all subjects, this ranged from a low of zero correctly identified tokens of a word pair, to a high of 16 correctly identified tokens. For the control subjects, only the first 6 correctly identified tokens of each word sequence were included in subsequent analyses.

The correctly identified stimuli were digitized by a VAX 11/780 pulse-code modulation system, using a 50 Hz low-pass filter and preemphasis on input, and a sampling rate of 10 KHz. The vowel-fricative(s)–vowel portion of each word pair was excised, and stimuli with a pause between words of greater than 1 sec were excluded (a total of 8 productions). Formant center-frequency and amplitude values for all remaining stimuli were determined at 10 ms intervals using a 28-term LPC model (cf. Markel & Gray, 1976).[2]

The following analysis frames were examined in detail:

1. The last sample window centered at least 10 ms before the offset of friction-free voicing for the first vowel.
2. The first sample window centered at least 10 ms after the onset of friction noise.
3. The sample window centered closest to the measured midpoint of friction duration.
4. The last sample window centered at least 10 ms before the offset of friction noise.
5. The first sample window centered at least 10 ms after the onset of friction-free voicing for the second vowel.

Center-frequency bandwidth and amplitude values of the second formant were calculated within the vocalic portions of the signal (measurement points 1 and 5). Formants with a bandwidth greater than 350 Hz were rejected. Spectral peaks within the friction noise were also determined (at measurement points 2, 3, and 4). These peaks were contiguous with the vowel's second formant and will hereafter be referred to as F2. In cases where the LPC techniques failed to determine F2 unambiguously, supplemental information was obtained from spectrograms produced on a Kay Sonograph.

RESULTS

The acoustic spectra were examined for evidence of anticipatory coarticulation of vowels with intervening fricatives. Separate ANOVAs were performed for 14 of the subjects examining the effects of first vowel (V1) identity

---

[2]The appropriateness of the LPC model for fricative analyses has been a subject of much recent debate. LPC assumes an all-pole model and may therefore make substantial errors when analyzing aperiodic sounds such as fricatives that contain zeros as well. Nevertheless, many studies have used LPC to study aperiodic sounds, with a good degree of similarity in the acoustic measures across studies. An additional consideration is that if LPC is thought to be appropriate for fricative analyses, the optimal number of LPC coefficients has yet to be specified. The data presented here were first analyzed using a 14-term model. The resulting spectra were highly similar to those of the 28-term model but with many more "holes" in which the analysis failed. Nevertheless, the statistical analyses showed the same pattern of results for spectra computed with the 14-term and 28-term models (see also Soli, 1981, Footnote 1).

(/i/ versus /u/), second vowel (V2) identity (/i/ versus /u/), and when possible fricative identity (/s/ versus /z#s/) on the second formant frequency determined at the five measurement points described above.[3] One nonfluent aphasic (NF2) produced so few correctly identified utterances that statistical treatment was not warranted. For this subject, only a qualitative description will be provided of trends in the acoustic spectra.

Fricative Effects

The effect of a word-final /z/ on formant frequency was first examined, although it was not a primary concern of the present study.

CONTROLS. Three control speakers (Cl, C4, and C5) showed lower F2 frequencies at measurement points 1–3, when the first word of the pair ended in /z/ rather than a vowel (F(1,40) ranged from 4.13 to 46.12, ps < .05). Two of these speakers (Cl and C5) also showed a significant interaction between the presence of a /z/ and the identity of the second vowel, when F2 was measured at V2 onset. Tukey's HSD showed that for both speakers, the difference in F2 frequency was greater between /Vz#si/ and /Vz#su/ than between /V#si/ and /V#su/ (ps < .05). The other two control speakers showed no main effects of fricative identity on formant frequency.

FLUENT APHASICS. Two fluent aphasic speakers (FL1 and FL2) showed effects of fricative identity on F2 measured at the friction midpoint (F(1,92) = 26.49, and F(1,66) = 21.92, ps < .001). In both cases, F2 was lower when /z/ was present. For two subjects (FL1 and FL4) the presence of the voiced fricative interacted with the identity of V2, measured at the offset of friction noise and the onset of V2 (FL1: F(1,92) = 10.27 and 8.22, respectively, ps < .01, FL2: F(1,54) = 6.58 and 5.35, respectively, ps < .05). Tukey's HSD showed that for FL1, the difference in F2 was greater for /Vz#si/ versus /Vz#su/ than for /V#si/ versus /V#su/; FL4 showed the opposite effect (ps < .05).

NONFLUENT APHASICS. None of the nonfluent aphasics showed an effect of fricative identity at any measurement point.

Anticipatory Vowel Effects

CONTROLS. The results for control subjects are presented in Figure 12-1. The ordinate shows the mean difference in F2 frequency between utterances with /i/ as the second vowel, and utterances with /u/ as the second vowel. Data for individual subjects (Cl thru C5) are plotted along the abscissa.

---

[3]Analysis of carryover coarticulation and fricative identity are reported in Tuller and Story (submitted for publication).

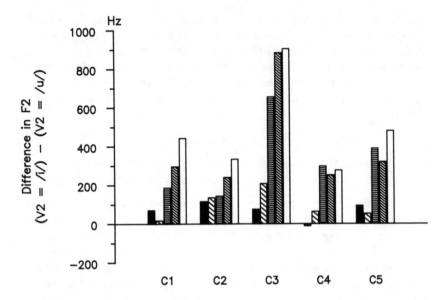

FIGURE 12-1. Anticipatory coarticulation (controls). The mean difference in F2 between utterances with /i/ as the second vowel and utterances with /u/ as the second vowel. Data for individual subjects are plotted along the abscissa for measurement point 1 (▬), 2 (▨), 3 (▥), 4 (▨), and 5 (▭).

The five columns for each subject represent the mean difference in F2 at measurement points 1 through 5, in order (see Figure 12-1 legend). ANOVAs computed for each subject revealed significant anticipatory effects of the second vowel for all subjects at least as early as the midpoint of friction noise (F(1,40) ranged from 9.01 to 150.69, ps < .01), that was consistent through the offset of friction noise and onset of the second vowel. One subject (C2) showed anticipation of the second vowel as early as the end of the first vowel (F(1,40) = 9.75, p < .01). Another subject (C4) showed acoustic evidence of anticipation beginning just after the onset of friction noise (F(1,40) - 5.51, p < .05). This subject also showed interactive anticipatory effects of V1 and V2 on the second formant frequency measured at friction onset (F(1,40) = 7.86, p < .01). Tukey's HSD revealed that V2 was anticipated as early as friction onset only when V1 = /u/.

FLUENT APHASICS. Figure 12-2 shows the mean difference in F2 values for utterances with V2 = /i/ versus V2 = /u/ spoken by fluent aphasic speakers. Axes and columns are as in Figure 12-1. A comparison of Figures 12-1 and 12-2 reveals that the controls and fluent aphasics performed in essentially identical fashion, with respect to both the extent and amount of anticipatory coarticulation. All 5 fluent aphasics showed anticipatory

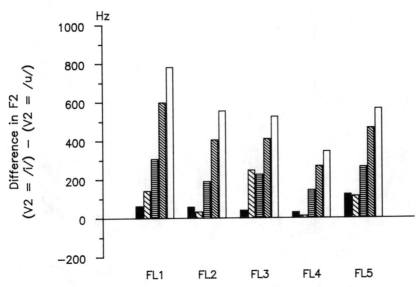

FIGURE 12-2. Anticipatory coarticulation (fluent aphasics).

effects of the second vowel at least as early as the midpoint of friction noise ($F(1,39\text{-}92)$)[4] ranged from 8.05 to 98.64 ps < .01). Two speakers, FL1 and FL3, showed anticipatory effects as early as friction onset ($F(1,92)$ = 7.37, $F(1,39)$ = 6.72, ps < .05) and a third speaker, FL5, showed significant anticipatory effects as early as the end of the first vowel ($F(1,53)$ = 13.98, p < .001).

NONFLUENT APHASICS. The 4 nonfluent aphasics whose productions were analyzed using ANOVA procedures showed a different pattern of anticipatory coarticulation than that evident for the controls' and fluent aphasics' productions. The mean F2 values for the 5 nonfluent aphasics are shown in Figure 12-3. Axes and columns are as in Figure 12-1.

Three nonfluent speakers (NF1, NF3, and NF5) showed significantly different F2 values as a function of the second vowel when F2 was measured just after the second vowel's onset (as one would expect, given that the vowel was correctly identified by listeners; ($F(1,34\text{-}69)$) ranged from 49.66 to 137.59, ps < .001). The same three speakers also produced significantly different F2 values for different upcoming vowels when F2 was measured just before the offset of friction noise ($F(1,34\text{-}69)$) ranged from 4.46 to 35.97, ps < .05). NF2, whose measured formant values were analyzed only qualitatively, also showed a tendency toward higher F2 values at the onset of the second vowel and the offset of friction noise, when the second vowel was /i/ rather then /u/. However, in contrast to the controls and fluent

---

[4]The aphasic speakers varied widely in the number of correctly produced words. Therefore, the range in the second term of the statistical degrees of freedom is presented as F(1, min-max).

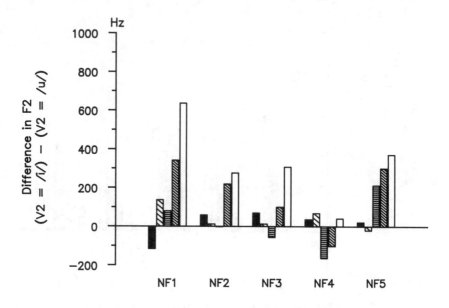

FIGURE 12-3. Anticipatory coarticulation (nonfluent aphasics).

aphasics only one of the 5 nonfluent aphasics (NF5) showed any influence of V2 as early as the friction midpoint (F(1,34) = 11.96, p < .01). NF4 showed a significant spectral effect at friction midpoint, but in the opposite direction: F2 for this speaker was consistently lower preceding /i/ than preceding /u/ (F(1,79) = 5.69, p < .05).

One possible explanation for the general lack of anticipatory coarticulation at friction midpoint for nonfluent speakers is that this measure might precede the "normal" onset of vowel anticipation. That is, nonfluent aphasic speakers tend to produce abnormally long segment durations (e.g., Kent & Rosenbek, 1983) so that friction midpoint relative to the upcoming vowel would be earlier for these speakers than for normal speakers and fluent aphasics. We decided to explore this possibility further, although two of the nonfluent speakers (NF2 and NF4) actually produced friction durations that were well within the normal range.

For the 4 nonfluent aphasic speakers who showed no evidence of anticipatory vowel articulation at friction midpoint, we determined spectral peaks within the friction noise for the sample window centered 70 ms before the onset of friction-free voicing for the second vowel. The choice of 70 ms had two motivations: (1) Katz (1987; see also chapter 11) reported preserved vowel anticipation in nonfluent productions measured 70 ms before vocalic voicing; and (2) 70 ms in almost all cases was temporally closer to the onset of vocalic voicing than was friction midpoint.

Separate 2 × 2 × 2 ANOVAs were performed for 3 nonfluent speakers examining the effects of first vowel identity, second vowel identity, and fricative identity on F2 measured 70 ms before V2 onset. As before, the remaining subjects' data (NF2) were analyzed only qualitatively. Two subjects (NF1 and NF3) showed a main effect of V2 on formant frequency (F(1, 33–70) = 20.64 and 14.07, respectively, ps < .001). No other main effect or interaction was significant for either subject. Subject NF4 again failed to show any anticipatory coarticulatory effect on F2 (F(1,73) = 2.61, p > .1). Subject NF2, whose measured formant values were analyzed only qualitatively did show some acoustic evidence of vowel anticipation, although it was not substantial. To summarize this analysis, when formant values were measured later in the friction noise, and thus closer to the second vowel, more subjects showed the spectral changes appropriate to the identity of the upcoming vowel.

DISCUSSION

The main finding of the present experiment is that some nonfluent aphasic speakers do not show acoustic anticipation of an upcoming vowel as early as do fluent aphasic speakers and normal controls. We want to stress that vowel anticipation is not *absent* in the nonfluent aphasics; 4 of the 5 speakers showed acoustic changes specific to the upcoming vowel, 70 ms prior to vocalic voicing. Rather, the acoustic consequences of anticipation may be delayed in the nonfluent aphasics, relative to normal. In contrast, the fact that the fluent aphasic speakers showed acoustic patterns that, like the control speakers, varied as early as friction midpoint as a function of upcoming vowel identity, suggests that the motoric deficits noted, for example, in the acoustic VOT analyses (Blumstein et al., 1977, 1980) are restricted to intrasegmental aspects of production.

Nevertheless these conclusions, like most others, are open to interpretation. In particular, they depend on what one defines as the "normal" extent of anticipatory processes—a question not yet resolved in the literature on "normal" speech production. For example, there is some evidence that the onset of a vowel's influence may be time-locked to the acoustic onset of the vocalic voicing (e.g., as suggested for example by Bell-Berti & Harris, 1979). Thus, to play the devil's advocate, it might be proposed that the only appropriate measure of vowel anticipation would be one taken a set number of milliseconds before voicing for the vowel begins (e.g., the "70 ms" measure). In fact, 4 of the 5 nonfluent aphasics tested showed appropriate vowel anticipation at that point. These data corroborate those of Katz (Chapter 11) from whom the 70 ms measure was derived.

At first blush, then, it appears that the literature dictates the choice of measurement point, that the measurement point should be defined by an absolute temporal interval, and that such a measure indicates essentially normal vowel anticipation by nonfluent aphasics. On closer inspection, however, it becomes apparent that this line of reasoning doesn't quite follow. Specifically, no current time-based theory of anticipatory coarticulation suggests that the absolute temporal extent of anticipation is the same across speakers. To the contrary, published evidence for time-locking is based on multiple speakers with little within-speaker temporal variation, but substantial across-speaker temporal variation (e.g., Bell-Berti & Harris, 1979; Gelfer, Bell-Berti, & Harris, 1980; Engstrand, 1981). Experiments on anticipatory coarticulation that do not necessarily support (or address) the time-locking issue also show substantial across-speaker temporal variation in anticipation, as well as anticipatory vowel effects that begin much earlier than 70 ms before the vowel. For example, Perkell (1986) reports that in productions of /isu/, forward lip movement for the /u/ occurs during the early portion of the /s/. Moreover, the one English speaker's data presented by Perkell (1986) shows that anticipatory lip protusion plateaus or peaks (i.e., is substantially complete) more than 125 ms before the end of the /s/ in all nine repetitions of /kasu/ (see also Daniloff & Moll, 1968). Similarly, for the nonfluent aphasics in this study who showed acoustic evidence of vowel anticipation 70 ms prior to friction-free voicing, the amount of spectral shift at that point was not markedly different from that measured 10 ms prior to friction-free voicing (see also Soli, 1981, for similar acoustic results). Identical results were reported by Katz (Chapter 11), who found no significant differences in the amount of coarticulatory shift measured 70 ms and 20 ms before the end of frication. For these reasons, we feel that the relative measure of friction midpoint is a more stringent test of the specific issue addressed in the present experiment than is the absolute 70 ms measure. Friction midpoint is close enough to vowel onset to allow vowel anticipation to be observed but not so close that anticipation would be substantially complete.

The present results are in close agreement with the small data set presented by Ziegler and von Cramon (1985, 1986a, 1986b). To our knowledge, however, the only source of detailed spectral information concerning coarticulatory patterns in aphasia, other than the present study, is provided by Katz (Chapter 11). Together, the two investigations provide a wealth of acoustic information not previously available and deserve closer scrutiny and comparison. In general, the present results and those of Katz are in agreement when analogous measures are considered. However, the possibility remains open for differences between Katz's data set and our own—differences that could further our understanding of anticipatory coarticulation in aphasia to a greater extent than could either experiment alone. For example, it could be asked whether Katz's nonfluent subjects show vowel anticipatory effects at friction midpoint. The perceptual results suggest they might not (as most of our nonfluent aphasics did not) because the overall perceptual scores for the nonfluent aphasics were lower than those for the normal subjects' stimuli when the entire fricative portion was excised and presented to listeners. In fact, most experiments showing that an upcoming vowel can be identified from the preceding fricative have used fricative stimuli of at least 150 ms duration (e.g., Kuehn & Moll, 1972; LaRiviere, Winitz, & Herriman, 1975; Repp & Mann, 1981; Yeni-Komshian & Soli, 1981). It may well be that for nonfluent aphasics' productions, perceptual testing of stimuli consisting of only the last 70 ms of frication would eliminate the perceptual advantage of the normals' productions.

On the other hand, Katz's nonfluent group may continue to show evidence of vowel anticipation as early as friction midpoint. This would, we feel, be an extremely interesting result. One basic difference between the two experiments is the structure of the stimuli. It may be that isolated fricative-vowel words allow for more extensive articulatory preposturing during the initial fricative than when the fricative-vowel is embedded in a word pair and is perhaps subject to greater temporal and spatial constraints.

The present investigation explored whether the acoustic consequences of anticipatory vowel articulation are present in the speech of control, nonfluent aphasic, and fluent aphasic speakers, measured at various points in time. The study was not designed to explore in detail the temporal extent of anticipatory articulatory gestures. Thus the lack of agreement between the present acoustic measures and the example of over-anticipation of velar movement reported by Itoh et al. (1979) is not too surprising. For example, our subjects could have begun articulatory anticipation of the vowel with an extremely low velocity gesture so that the acoustic consequences of the gesture were not apparent until some time later. Similarly, in Itoh et al.'s (1979) example of a required production of [deeneedesu] that was produced as [deedeedesu], the onset of velar lowering occurred at a time appropriate for the required utterance, but with a markedly decreased velocity of lowering. When the tongue tip constricted the oral cavity for production of /n/, the velum was not yet low enough to allow the airflow through the nasal cavity. The point is that the actual trajectory of articulatory movements, not simply the time of movement onset, will influence when the acoustic and perceptual consequences of the gesture are observable.

In conclusion, we want to stress that the observed disruption of the acoustic consequences of anticipatory coarticulation in some nonfluent aphasic speakers occurred in utterances that were perceived as phonemically correct. One implication is that the acoustically abnormal coarticulatory pattern may contribute to our perception of speech produced by nonfluent aphasics as being "effortful" or "labored." Moreover, some so-called phonemic errors common in nonfluent aphasia, such as schwa insertion and vowel diphthongization, might also be accounted for as more extreme disruptions in the interarticulator spatiotemporal patterns. It is our intention to proceed, as far as possible, in trying to understand the error patterns in aphasic speech in terms of the coordination of motor speech events and their acoustic and perceptual consequences.

ACKNOWLEDGMENTS

This work was supported by NINCDS grants NS-17778 to Cornell University Medical Center, NS-13617 to Haskins Laboratories, and by the Ariel and Benjamin Lowin Medical Research Foundation (administered through the Stuttering Center, Baylor College of Medicine).

REFERENCES

Alajouanine, T., Ombredane, A., & Durand, M. (1939). *Le syndrome de la desintegration phonetique dans l'aphasie.* Paris: Masson.

Bell-Berti, F., & Harris, K.S. (1979). Anticipatory coarticulation: Some implications from a study of lip rounding. *Journal of the Acoustical Society of America, 65,* 1268–1270.

Blumstein, S.E. (1973). *A phonological investigation of aphasic speech.* The Hague: Mouton.

Blumstein, S.E., Cooper, W.E., Goodglass, H., Statlender, S., & Gottlieb, J. (1980). Production deficits in aphasia: A voice-onset time analysis. *Brain and Language, 9,* 153–170.

Blumstein, S.E., Cooper, W. D., Zurif, E. B., & Caramazza, A. (1977). The perception and production of voice-onset-time in aphasia. *Neuropsychologia, 15,* 371–383.

Buckingham, H.W. (1981). Explanations for the concept of apraxia of speech. In M. Sarno (Ed.), *Acquired aphasia.* New York: Academic Press.

Collins, M., Rosenbek, J., & Wertz, R. (1983). Spectrographic analysis of vowel and word duration in apraxia of speech. *Journal of Speech and Hearing Research, 26,* 224–230.

Daniloff, R.G., & Moll, K.L. (1968). Coarticulation of lip-rounding. *Journal of Speech and Hearing Research, 11,* 707–721.

Darley, F.L., Aronson, A.E., & Brown, J.R. (1975). *Motor speech disorders.* Philadelphia: W.B. Saunders.

Duffy, J.R., & Gawle, C.A. (1984). Apraxic speakers' vowel duration in consonant-vowel-consonant syllables. In J. Rosenbek, M.R. McNeil, & A.E. Aronson (Eds.), *Apraxia of speech.* San Diego: College-Hill Press.

Elman, J., & McClelland, J. (1983). Speech perception as a cognitive process: The interactive activation model. ICS Report No. 8302. San Diego: University of California, Institute of Cognitive Science.

Engstrand, 0. (1981). Acoustic constraints of invariant input representation? An experimental study of selected articulatory movements and targets. *Reports from Uppsala University Department of Linguistics, 7,* 67–94.

Engstrand, O. (1983). *Articulatory coordination in selected VCV utterances: A means-end view* (Unpublished doctoral dissertation, Department of Linguistics, University of Uppsala, Uppsala, Sweden).

Freeman, F.J., Sands, E.S., & Harris, K.S. (1978). Temporal coordination of phonation and articulation in a case of verbal apraxia: A voice onset time study. *Brain and Language, 6,* 106–111.

Gandour, J., & Dardarananda, R. (1984). Voice onset time in aphasia: Thai, II. Production. *Brain and Language, 23,* 177–205.

Gelfer, C. E., Bell-Berti, F., & Harris, K.S. (1985). Determining the extent of coarticulation: Effects of experimental design. In *Haskins Laboratories Status Reports on Speech Research SR-82/83,* 19–31.

Goodglass, H., & Kaplan, E. (1972). *The assessment of aphasia and related disorders.* Philadelphia: Lea and Febiger.

Hockett, C. (1955). *Manual of phonology.* Publications in Anthropology and Linguistics (No. 11). Bloomington, IN: Indiana University Press.

Hoit-Dalgaard, J., Murry, T., & Kopp, H.G. (1983). Voice onset time production and perception in apraxic subjects. *Brain and Language, 20,* 329–339.

Hughes, G.M., & Halle, M. (1956). Spectral properties of fricative consonants. *Journal of the Acoustical Society of America, 28,* 303–310.

Itoh, M., Sasanuma, S., Hirose, H., Yoshioka, H., & Ushijima, T. (1980). Abnormal articulatory dynamics in a patient with apraxia of speech: X-Ray microbeam observation. *Brain and Language, 11,* 66–75.

Itoh, M., Sasanuma, S., Tatsumi, I.F., Murakami, S., Fukusako, Y., & Suzuki, T. (1982). Voice onset time characteristics in apraxia of speech. *Brain and Language, 17,* 193–210.

Itoh, M., Sasanuma, S., & Ushijima, T. (1979). Velar movement during speech in a patient with apraxia of speech. *Brain and Language, 7,* 227–240.

Jassem, W. (1964). The formant patterns of fricative consonants. *Language and Speech, 7,* 15–31.

Katz, W. (1987). An acoustic and perceptual investigation of anticipatory coarticulation in aphasia (Unpublished Ph.D. dissertation, Brown University).

Kent, R.D. (1976). Models of speech production. In N.J. Lass (Ed.), *Contemporary issues in experimental phonetics.* New York: Academic Press.

Kent, R.D., & Rosenbek, J.C. (1983). Acoustic patterns of apraxia of speech. *Journal of Speech and Hearing Research, 26,* 231–249.

Kuehn, D.P., & Moll, L.K. (1972). Perceptual effects of forward coarticulation. *Journal of Speech and Hearing Research, 15,* 654–664.

LaRiviere, C., Winitz, H., & Herriman, E. (1975). The distribution of perceptual cues in English prevocalic fricatives. *Journal of Speech and Hearing Research, 18,* 613–622.

Lisker, L., & Abramson, A.S. (1967). Some effects of context on voice onset time in English stops. *Language and Speech, 10,* 1–28.

Luria, A.R. (1966). *Higher cortical functions in man.* New York: Basic Books.

MacKay, D. (1970). Spoonerisms: The structure of errors in the serial order of speech. *Neuropsychologia, 8,* 823–850.

MacNeilage, P.F. (1980). Speech production. *Language and Speech, 23,* 3–23

MacNeilage, P.F., Hutchinson, J., & Lasater, S. (1981). The production of speech: Development and dissolution of motoric and premotoric processes. In J. Long & A. Baddeley (Eds.), *Attention and performance IX.* Hillsdale, NJ: Erlbaum, pp. 503–519.

MacNeilage, P., & Ladefoged, P. (1976). The production of speech and language. In E.C. Carterette & M.P. Friedman (Eds.), *Handbook of perception: Language and speech.* New York: Academic Press.

Markel, J.D., & Gray, A.H. (1976). *Linear prediction of speech.* Berlin: Springer-Verlag.

Marquardt, T., Rinehart, J., & Peterson, H. (1979). Markedness analysis of phonemic substitution errors in apraxia of speech. *Journal of Communication Disorders, 12,* 481–494.

McGarr, N.S., & Harris, K.S. (1983). Articulatory control in a deaf speaker. In I. Hochberg, H. Levitt, & M.J. Osberger (Eds.), *Speech of the hearing impaired: Research, training and personnel preparation.* Baltimore, MD: University Park Press, pp. 75–95.

McGarr, N.S., Kobayashi, N., & Honda, K. (1984). Electromyographic and kinematic measures of articulatory coordination in a deaf speaker. *Journal of the Acoustical Society of America, 74*(Abstract), S23.

Perkell, J.S. (1986). Coarticulation strategies: Preliminary implications of a detailed analysis of lower lip protrusion movements. *Speech Communication, 5,* 47–68.

Repp, B.H., & Mann, V.A. (1981). Perceptual assessment of fricative-stop coarticulation. *Journal of the Acoustical Society of America, 69,* 1154–1163.

Ryalls, J.H. (1981). Motor aphasia: Acoustic correlates of phonetic disintegration in vowels. *Neuropsychologia, 19,* 365–374.

Shankweiler, D.P., & Harris, K.S. (1966). An experimental approach to the problem of articulation in aphasia. *Cortex, 2,* 277–292.

Shankweiler, D., Harris, K.S., & Taylor, M.L. (1968). Electromyographic studies of articulation in aphasia. *Archives of Physical Medicine and Rehabilitation, 49,* 1–8.

Shewan, C., Leeper, H., & Booth (1984). An analysis of voice onset time (VOT) in aphasic and normal subjects. In J. Rosenbek, M.R. McNeil, & A.E. Aronson (Eds.), *Apraxia of speech.* San Diego, CA: College-Hill Press.

Soli, S. (1981). Second formants in fricatives: Acoustic consequences of fricative-vowel coarticulation. *Journal of the Acoustical Society of America, 70,* 976–984.

Tuller, B. (1984). On categorizing aphasic speech errors. *Neuropsychologia, 22,* 547–557.

Tuller, B., & Story, R. (1986). Co-articulation in aphasic speech. *Journal of the Acoustical Society of America (Suppl. 1), 80,* MM17.

Tuller, B. & Story, R. (Submitted for publication). Anticipatory and carryover coarticulation in aphasia: An acoustic study.

Williams, S.E., & Seaver, E.J. (1986). A comparison of speech sound durations in three syndromes of aphasia. *Brain and Language, 29,* 171–182.

Yeni-Komshian, G., & Soli, S.D. (1981). Recognition of vowels from information in fricatives: Perceptual evidence of fricative-vowel coarticulation. *Journal of the Acoustical Society of America, 70,* 966–975.

Ziegler, W., & von Cramon, D. (1985). Anticipatory coarticulation in a patient with apraxia of speech. *Brain and Language, 26,* 117–130.

Ziegler, W., & von Cramon, D. (1986a). Disturbed coarticulation in apraxia of speech: Acoustic evidence. *Brain and Language, 29,* 34–47.

Ziegler, W., & von Cramon, D. (1986b). Timing deficits in apraxia of speech. *European Archives of Psychiatry and Neurological Sciences, 236,* 44–49.

AUTHOR INDEX

S U B J E C T   I N D E X

Acoustic analysis methods in phonetic
  realization of phonological
  contrasts in aphasic patients,
  166–167
Acoustic experiment in anticipatory
  labial and lingual coarticulation
  in aphasia
analysis, 225–228
results, 228–229, 230–232(t), 233
stimuli, 225
subjects, 224–225
Acoustic and perceptual data,
  correlation between, 235–236
Affective arena in informational
  processing model, definition of,
  181–182, 183, 188
Alveolar fricative in
  electropalatographic
  investigations, 120
tongue-palate contacts, 124(f)
Alveolar stops and nasals in
  electropalatographic
  investigations, 119
tongue-palate contacts, 120(f), 121(f),
  122(f), 123(f)
Amplitude
as acoustic parameter, 81
and tone production in aphasia, 45
Anticipatory coarticulation in aphasia,
  investigation of
discussion, 255–258
method
  data analysis, 249–250
  procedure, 248–249
  stimuli, 248
  subjects, 247–248, 249(t)
results, 250–251
  anticipatory vowel effects, 251–255
  fricative effects, 251
speech production, view of, 243
studies on, 245–247
voice-onset time patterning, 245
Anticipatory labial and lingual
  coarticulation in aphasia, 222–224

acoustic experiment
analysis, 225–228
results, 228–229, 233
stimuli, 225
subjects, 224–225
correlation between acoustic and
  perceptual data, 235–236
discussion, 236–239
perceptual experiment
procedures, 233
results, 233, 235
Aphasia
anticipatory. See Anticipatory labial
  and lingual coarticulation, in
  aphasia
coarticulation in, 222–224
consonant production in. See
  Consonant production deficits
  in aphasia
subjects, descriptive data for, 249(t)
tone production in. See Tone
  production in aphasia
vowel production in. See Vowel
  production in aphasia
Aphasic errors, classification of
discussion, 176–177
examples, 168–175
investigations, 163–166
methods, 166–167
Aphasic patients, investigation of
  anticipatory velocities in
discussion, 155, 157–159
method
  data analysis, 140–141
  procedure, 138–139
  speech materials, 139–140
  subjects, 137–138
results, 141, 144–145, 146–147, 150,
  151, 154
summary of, 160–161
Aphasic patients, intonation in. See
  Intonation in aphasic patients
Apraxia Battery for Adults (ABA), 196,
  197(t), 198

267

N O T E S

N O T E S

N O T E S

N O T E S